Arthritis

Your Complete Exercise Guide

The Cooper Clinic and Research Institute Fitness Series

Neil F. Gordon, MD, PhD, MPH
The Cooper Institute for Aerobics Research
Dallas, Texas

Human Kinetics Publishers

In memory of Raymond Salmon,
who first showed me that it is possible to remain courageous
despite a rampant case of rheumatoid arthritis.

Library of Congress Cataloging-in-Publication Data

Gordon, Neil F.
　　Arthritis : your complete exercise guide / Neil F. Gordon.
　　　　p.　cm. -- (The Cooper Clinic and Research Institute fitness
　　series)
　　Includes bibliographical references and index.
　　ISBN 0-87322-392-6
　　1. Arthritis--Exercise therapy.　I. Title.　II. Series.
　　RC933.G625　1993
　　616.7'22062--dc20　　　　　　　　　　　　　　　92-6294
　　　　　　　　　　　　　　　　　　　　　　　　　　　　CIP

ISBN: 0-87322-392-6

Copyright © 1993 by Neil F. Gordon

Notice: Exercise and health are matters that vary necessarily between individuals. Readers should speak with their own doctors about their individual needs *before* starting any exercise program. This book is *not* intended as a substitute for the medical advice and supervision of your personal physician. Any application of the recommendations set forth in the following pages is at the reader's discretion and sole risk.

Human Kinetics books are available at special discounts for bulk purchase for sales promotions, premiums, fund-raising, or educational use. Special editions or book excerpts can also be created to specification. For details, contact the Special Sales Manager at Human Kinetics.

Printed in the United States of America

10　9　8　7　6　5　4　3　2　1

Human Kinetics Publishers
Box 5076, Champaign, IL 61825-5076
1-800-747-4457

Europe Office:
Human Kinetics Publishers (Europe) Ltd.
P.O. Box IW14
Leeds LS16 6TR
England
0532-781708

Canada Office:
Human Kinetics Publishers
P.O. Box 2503, Windsor, ON N8Y 4S2
1-800-465-7301 (in Canada only)

Australia Office:
Human Kinetics Publishers
P.O. Box 80
Kingswood 5062
South Australia
374-0433

Contents

Foreword

Each book in The Cooper Clinic and Research Institute Fitness Series covers an exercise rehabilitation program devised to help Cooper Clinic patients and other patients around the world recover from a chronic disorder. The series covers diabetes, chronic fatigue, breathing problems, stroke, and arthritis.

I anticipate that the readers of this arthritis book will be highly motivated fighters—people who aren't going to let their malady, painful though it may sometimes be, get the best of them. They're going to do what needs to be done to fight back and win! If you fall into this category, you've got the right book in your hands, for I believe my staff at The Cooper Aerobics Center* and I have developed one of the finest—and safest—arthritis exercise rehabilitation programs.

Although arthritis doesn't often make the headlines like heart disease, cancer, or AIDS, it's nonetheless a ubiquitous health problem, often profoundly burdensome. The statistical facts about arthritis are startling: One in every seven Americans has it—that's an estimated

---

*The Cooper Aerobics Center, founded by Ken Cooper in Dallas in the early 1970s, is comprised of the Cooper Clinic, a preventive and rehabilitative medicine facility; The Cooper Institute for Aerobics Research, where researchers study the role of exercise and other lifestyle factors in the maintenance of health; the Cooper Wellness Program, which provides a supportive, live-in environment where participants can focus time and attention on the challenging task of how to make positive lifestyle changes; and the Cooper Fitness Center, a health club in which all members' exercise efforts are supervised by a well-trained staff of health professionals.

14.3% of the population of the United States! One in every three families in the country has a member with arthritis. Most people associate arthritis with the elderly, so it probably won't surprise you to learn that the prevalence (the number of people with arthritis at any one time) increases with age. Almost half of all Americans 65 years or older are seriously debilitated by an arthritic condition. And the middle-aged are not immune. About 28% of Americans between 45 and 64 years of age also have arthritis, as do a fairly sizable portion of even younger adults. No, arthritis is not simply a disease of the aged.

Whether an arthritis patient is young or old, the potential hardships are similar. A severe case of arthritis can result in staggering medical expenses. Arthritis causes pain, suffering for many, and sometimes total incapacity, turning some patients into premature invalids. In addition there are a host of human relations problems such a debilitating state of affairs can trigger.

One of the worst things about arthritis is its negative effect on quality of life. Even a moderate case of arthritis can destroy a person's ability to be productive and fully functional. *Arthritis causes more missed days of work and inability to fulfill daily activities than any other well-known chronic condition.* When you compare the debilitating impact of arthritis to that of acute or short-term conditions, arthritis is still near the top; it's second after acute respiratory conditions, such as the common cold and influenza.

Exercise, in particular aerobic exercise, is not emphasized enough in the arthritis treatment books already on the market, and so we felt it necessary to write this one. What this book offers that most others don't is comprehensive, state-of-the-art advice on how an arthritis patient should go about starting an exercise program, including information about how much exercise is enough to improve your health.

Anyone familiar with my books knows that I believe people need all the motivation they can get to break a bad health habit and replace it with a good one. To provide you with a strong incentive to maintain your health through regular exertion while avoiding the aspects of exercise that are risky for arthritis patients, this book comes complete with a Health Points System. The system is designed to keep you exercising over the long haul. It will ease you into a healthier lifestyle and motivate you to persevere even on those days when you feel most tempted to backslide.

It's my hope that this book will serve as a springboard for discussions about exercise between you and your doctor. I also hope it will make you more self-sufficient for the small details involved in working exercise into your daily routine. On the other hand, I don't ever want you to regard the advice as a substitute for that of your doctor or any other health-care practitioner familiar with your case.

Arthritis management has come a long way over the years. Today arthritis patients can be rehabilitated and given the tools, one of which is exercise, to exert more control over this problem than ever before. After reading this book, most of you will discover that you can partially—or almost fully—reverse many of the disabilities your arthritis has caused and, thus, return to a more active lifestyle. Cheer up. You really do have far more control over arthritis than you ever thought possible!

Kenneth H. Cooper, MD, MPH

About the Author

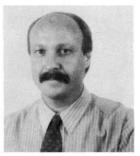

D r. Neil F. Gordon is widely regarded as a leading medical authority on exercise and health. Before receiving his master's degree in public health from the University of California at Los Angeles in 1989, Dr. Gordon received doctoral degrees in exercise physiology and medicine at the University of the Witwatersrand in Johannesburg, South Africa. He also served as medical director of cardiac rehabilitation and exercise physiology for 6 years at I Military Hospital in Pretoria, South Africa.

Since 1987, Dr. Gordon has been the director of exercise physiology at the internationally renowned Cooper Institute for Aerobics Research in Dallas, Texas. He has also written over 50 papers on exercise and medicine.

Dr. Gordon is a member of the American Heart Association and American Diabetes Association. He is a fellow of the American College of Sports Medicine and the American Association of Cardiovascular and Pulmonary Rehabilitation. He also has served on the board of directors for AACVPR, the Texas Association of Cardiovascular and Pulmonary Rehabilitation, and the American Heart Association (Dallas affiliate).

Preface

A ny series of books as comprehensive as The Cooper Clinic and Research Institute Fitness Series is likely to have an interesting story behind it, and this one certainly does. Our story began over a decade ago, shortly after I completed my medical training. Because of my keen interest in sports medicine (which was why I went to medical school in the first place), I volunteered to help establish an exercise rehabilitation program for patients with chronic diseases at a major South African hospital. To get the ball rolling I decided to telephone patients who had recently been treated at the hospital. My very first call planted the seed for writing a series of books that would (a) educate patients with chronic medical conditions about the many benefits of a physically active lifestyle and (b) lead them step-by-step down the road to improved health.

That telephone call was an eye-opener for me, a relative novice in the field of rehabilitation medicine. The patient, a middle-aged man who had recently suffered a heart attack, bellowed into the phone: "Why are you trying to create more problems for me? Isn't it enough that I've been turned into an invalid for the rest of my life by a heart attack?" Fortunately I kept my cool and convinced him to give the program a try—after all, what did he have to lose? Within months he was "miraculously" transformed into a man with a new zest for life. Like the thousands of men and women with chronic disorders with whom I've subsequently worked in South Africa and, more recently, the United States, he had experienced first-hand the numerous physical and psychological benefits of a medically prescribed exercise rehabilitation program.

Today it's known that a comprehensive exercise rehabilitation program, such as the one outlined in this book, is an essential component of state-of-the-art medical care for patients with a variety of chronic conditions, including arthritis. But, despite the many benefits unfolding through numerous research studies, patients with chronic medical conditions are usually not much better informed than that heart patient was prior to my telephone call. This book is meant to help fill this void for persons with arthritis by providing you with practical, easy-to-follow information about exercise rehabilitation for use in collaboration with your doctor.

To accomplish this I've set out this book as follows. In chapter 1 you'll meet two of our arthritis patients. Their stories are intended to introduce you to some basic concepts about arthritis, exercise, and rehabilitation. In chapter 2 you'll discover the wonderful benefits of a physically active lifestyle. Toward the end of this chapter I do temper my obvious enthusiasm for exercise by pointing out some of its potential risks for persons with arthritis. In chapter 3 I'll show you, step-by-step, how to embark on a sensible exercise rehabilitation program. In chapter 4 you'll learn how to use the Health Points System to determine precisely how much exercise you need to optimize your health and fitness, without exerting yourself to the point where exercise can become risky. At the end of this chapter I'll give you some useful tips for sticking with your exercise program once you've begun. Finally, in chapter 5, I provide you with essential safety guidelines. Although exercise is a far more normal state for the human body than being sedentary, I want you to keep your risk—however small it may be—as low as possible.

View the programs in this book as prototypes. It is up to you and your doctor to make changes in these prototypes—that is, to adapt my programs—to suit the medical realities of your specific case of arthritis. Set realistic goals for yourself. Above all remember that no book can remove the need for close supervision by a patient's own doctor.

By the time you have completed this book, I hope that you'll have renewed hope for a healthier, longer, more enjoyable life. If you then act on the advice and adopt a more physically active lifestyle, this book will have supplemented the efforts of the Arthritis Foundation in the United States and other similar organizations around the world in the battle against arthritis. If it does, the time spent preparing *Arthritis: Your Complete Exercise Guide* will have been well worth the effort.

Neil F. Gordon, MD, PhD, MPH

Acknowledgments

To prepare a series of books as comprehensive and complex as this, I have required the assistance and cooperation of many talented people. To adequately acknowledge all would be impossible. However, I would be remiss not to recognize a few special contributions.

Ken Cooper, MD, MPH, chairman and founder of the Cooper Clinic, was of immense assistance in initiating this series. In addition to writing the introduction and providing many useful suggestions, he continues to serve as an inspiration to me and millions of people around the world.

Larry Gibbons, MD, MPH, medical director of the Cooper Clinic, co-authored with me *The Cooper Clinic Cardiac Rehabilitation Program*. In doing so he made an invaluable contribution to many of the concepts used in this series, especially the Health Points System.

Jacqueline Thompson, a talented writer based in Staten Island, New York, provided excellent editorial assistance with the first draft of this series. Her contributions and those of Herb Katz, a New York–based literary agent, greatly enhanced the practical value of this series.

Charles Sterling, EdD, executive director of The Cooper Institute for Aerobics Research, provided much needed guidance and support while working on this series, as did John Duncan, PhD; Chris Scott,

MS; Pat Brill, PhD; Kia Vaandrager, MS; Conrad Earnest, MS; and my many other colleagues at The Cooper Aerobics Center.

James Fries, MD, a world-renowned authority in the field of arthritis from Stanford University, reviewed the first draft of *Arthritis: Your Complete Exercise Guide* and provided many excellent suggestions.

My thanks to Rainer Martens, president of Human Kinetics Publishers, without whom this series could not have been published. Rainer, Holly Gilly (my developmental editor), and other staff members at Human Kinetics Publishers did a fantastic job in making this series a reality. It was a pleasurable and gratifying experience to work with them.

A special thanks to the patients who allowed me to tell their stories and to all my patients over the years from whom I have learned so much about exercise and rehabilitation.

Finally I want to thank my wonderful family—my wife, Tracey, and daughters, Kim and Terri—for their patience, support, and understanding in preparing this series.

To all these people, and the many others far too numerous to list, many thanks for making this book a reality and in so doing benefiting arthritis patients around the world.

Credits

Developmental Editor—Holly Gilly; *Managing Editor*—Moyra Knight; *Assistant Editors*—Valerie Hall, John Wentworth, Laura Bofinger; *Copyeditor*—Mary Rose Cottingham; *Proofreader*—Pam Johnson; *Indexer*—Sheila Ary; *Production Director*—Ernie Noa; *Text Design*—Keith Blomberg; *Text Layout*—Sandra Meier, Kathy Fuoss, Tara Welsch; *Cover Design*—Jack Davis; *Factoids*—Doug Burnett; *Technique Drawings*—Tim Offenstein; *Interior Art*—Kathy Fuoss, Gretchen Walters; *Printer*—United Graphics

The Cooper Clinic and Research Institute Fitness Series

Arthritis: *Your Complete Exercise Guide*

Breathing Disorders: *Your Complete Exercise Guide*

Chronic Fatigue: *Your Complete Exercise Guide*

Diabetes: *Your Complete Exercise Guide*

Stroke: *Your Complete Exercise Guide*

Chapter 1

Moving Beyond the Pain of Arthritis

Arthritis is the most democratic of the world's diseases. If you develop it, you are in company with 37 million other people in the United States alone. Worldwide it touches the lives of close to 1 billion people. Although its origins are still unknown, one thing is perfectly clear—no adult is immune from the threat of its aches and pains. Those affected are rich and poor, young and old, obscure and famous.

Compared with contracting other diseases, getting arthritis may not seem that devastating. It's not a communicable disease like AIDS or tuberculosis. Unlike heart disease and cancer, arthritis is usually not a direct cause of death, although death can occur in severe cases of certain types of arthritis. Rather, arthritis is often little more than annoying. Unfortunately what starts out as an annoyance often turns into a major debilitator if steps, like those outlined in this book, aren't taken to manage the arthritis properly and retard, perhaps even reverse, its progression. Indeed there are few—if any—diseases more incapacitating than a rampant case of arthritis.

One person who didn't let premature arthritis hold her back was world-renowned tennis pro Billie Jean King.[1] At age 18 years, she rammed both knees into a dashboard during a car accident. Five

1

years later her doctor told her she had developed osteoarthritis as a consequence. Today, 25 years after that accident, Billie Jean King is retired from an incredible athletic career distinguished by 20 Wimbledon titles, 4 U.S. Open singles championships, and singles titles in both the French and Australian Grand Slam championships. But she still follows a daily exercise regimen to keep her arthritis in check, just as she did during the heyday of her tennis career.

"Back in the 1960s when I was diagnosed, most physicians didn't know much about arthritis rehabilitation," Billie Jean recalls ruefully. She was given a namby-pamby exercise rehabilitation program. Instinctively Billie Jean knew it wouldn't do much to foster recuperation from the knee operations she'd undergone. Instead she developed her own "very active" athletic training schedule that included concentrated muscle-strengthening exercises—particularly to build up the muscles around her knees—and aerobic exercise training. Looking back, she estimates it took her about a year after each operation to regain top form.

Like your arthritis, Billie Jean King's may never go away completely. But she has learned to live with it. "What are you going to do—stop living and stop performing? No way. You simply have to keep going. Sadly, I see too many arthritic patients who are afraid to exercise." From her own experience, Billie Jean thinks this is a mistake. "When I don't exercise, I feel worse. It's that simple." Her advice is this: "Consult your physician, preferably one who is knowledgeable about rehabilitation—and then start an on-going exercise program. You'll be surprised how well exercise works for the mind as well as the body!"

The success of Billie Jean King and others like her is a testament to the fact that *you can lead an active lifestyle despite arthritis*. The exercise rehabilitation program I outline is one of your keys to staying energetic and involved in life and all the promise it still holds for you. Indeed it's regular exercise at our Cooper Fitness Center that is partly responsible for the wonderful recuperation of two people you're about to meet.

CASE HISTORY OF ALAN HOFFMAN

Two years ago, Alan Hoffman, a 53-year-old dentist, went to his doctor for a routine annual checkup, complaining of chronic pain in his right hand and left hip. The pain in his joints wasn't new, he admitted, but he'd stoically endured it for years because the aching was intermittent. Now it was turning into an everyday occurrence, and he was worried. As a dentist, he stood on his feet for hours every day; and, to make things worse, he was right-handed. How could he continue to make a living if his hip and hand gave out on him?

Alan was moderately overweight, and his doctor could easily see that a weight-bearing joint like his hip might be crying out for relief. Twenty pounds (9 kilograms) or so less body weight, hence less stress on the painful hip joint, would certainly be a step in the right direction. But clearly there was more to Alan's problem than mere excess poundage. Alan's doctor examined his joints, X-rayed them, and took blood tests, all the while inquiring at length about Alan's lifestyle and medical history.

The results, particularly of the X rays, revealed osteoarthritis, but the doctor could find no readily identifiable cause, meaning Alan had *primary osteoarthritis*. (Another form, called *secondary osteoarthritis*, results from such predisposing factors as specific joint trauma, usually injuries, and certain diseases.[2] Billie Jean King's arthritis is a perfect example of secondary osteoarthritis.)

Yes, arthritis is a chronic condition, Alan's doctor explained, but the doctor had several ideas about how to relieve Alan's painful symptoms to the point where they would be unlikely to interfere with his livelihood. First, his doctor prescribed medication to relieve the joint pain and any inflammation that might be present. Next, the doctor referred Alan to our Cooper Fitness Center for exercise therapy and a weight loss program.

On Alan's arrival at the center, he was in class 2 of the functional capacity classification scheme presented in chapter 2 (page 15). In the intervening year and a half, he's lost 25 pounds. He eats more selectively and works out faithfully, both at home and at the center. At home, Alan does stretching exercises and strength training, followed by a stint on a stationary bike while he's watching the news. He likes the bike because its design works arms and legs simultaneously.

During his first year as a Cooper Fitness Center member, Alan used brisk walking in the winter and swimming in the summer to supplement his home stationary cycling and to earn his recommended weekly quota of 100 health points. Alan has also recently embarked on a more serious muscle strengthening program. Twice each week now, after cooling down from his walk or swim, he tackles the resistance training machines at the center.

Alan still has some joint stiffness in the morning and his pain recurs occasionally, but it's much better. He used to wake up with his left hip joint so stiff he limped for about 10 minutes before he could walk

Case History, Alan Hoffman

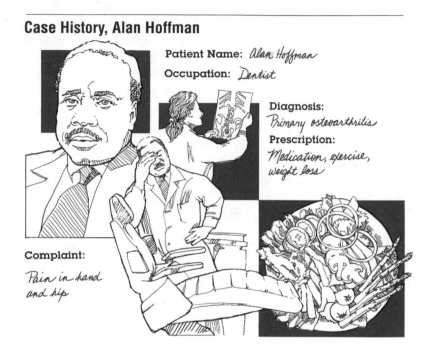

Patient Name: *Alan Hoffman*

Occupation: *Dentist*

Diagnosis:
Primary osteoarthritis

Prescription:
Medication, exercise, weight loss

Complaint:
Pain in hand and hip

properly. Now his hip joint might feel a little stiff as he slings his legs over the side of the bed to get up, but walking energetically to the bathroom is no longer something he has to think about. Today Alan takes pain medication only on those rare occasions when his joints really act up.

Alan readily admits that the linchpin of his recovery is faithful adherence to regular exercise. He calls exercise a "miracle cure," though not in the usual sense of its being instantaneous or making a disease disappear forever. "Exercise requires perseverance and time to work its magic. But it does eventually work wonders," says Alan. The miracle it worked for him was to increase his aerobic fitness (which we measure at the Cooper Clinic via treadmill exercise testing) by 30% and his strength by almost 60%. His blood-lipid profile is also much improved; though this doesn't affect his arthritis, Alan is pleased, because heart disease runs in his family.

CASE HISTORY OF CHERYL LEWIS

Cheryl Lewis, 48, is another convert to using regular exercise to control a moderately severe case of *rheumatoid arthritis*, another type.

Three years ago, Cheryl started to develop mild pain in her joints on both sides of her body. Her knuckles, middle joints of her fingers, wrists, elbows, knees, and ankles all bothered her to some extent as she went about her daily household chores.

Over a period of 3 months, the pain began to worsen, but that was not Cheryl's only problem. Her mental state was deteriorating even faster. The fear of developing a severe case of arthritis, like the one that had made an invalid of her father, was beginning to paralyze Cheryl. The picture of him sitting idly in his favorite rocking chair by the kitchen window, day in and day out, began to haunt her thoughts. He had developed such bad arthritis before age 50 that he'd been forced to quit work and live on disability insurance. Cheryl was too frightened to see her own doctor and find out if she was destined to follow in her father's footsteps. Instead she endured her aches and pains in silence, hoping that she'd wake up one day to discover it was all a bad dream.

Instead of awakening from a bad dream, Cheryl began awakening in the morning with a body that was stiff all over. It took about 2 hours before her stiff joints would loosen up. Not only that, her joints were often swollen and warm to the touch. And she was having a hard time coping with her usual housework. She tired more easily and, for the first time in her life, was losing weight without trying.

Cheryl's husband noticed the changes and insisted she see the family doctor for a checkup. It didn't take Cheryl's doctor long to confirm her worst fears. Yes, her father's nemesis was also hers. Although there was still no cure for rheumatoid arthritis, her physician explained, treatment of the disease had come a long way since the time her father suffered from it, 30 years earlier. There was a reasonably good chance she could still lead an active, productive life by adhering to a special treatment and rehabilitation program; he referred her to a specialist, called a *rheumatologist*.

Cheryl's rheumatologist was even more optimistic. She immediately put her on medications to alleviate the pain, stiffness, and swelling and monitored her progress closely for months, modifying her drug therapy according to her response to it. Once Cheryl started to feel better physically and stopped her mental brooding, she moved into the second phase—a comprehensive rehabilitation program that included physical as well as occupational therapy. The rheumatologist also encouraged her to join the Arthritis Foundation to meet others with her condition and to learn more about the disease and treatments. (For information about the foundation and its many outstanding services, contact your local chapter or write to Arthritis Foundation, P.O. Box 19000, Atlanta, GA 30326, United States.)

About 18 months after the first onset of symptoms, Cheryl had reached the happy state in which her condition was no longer active: The arthritis wasn't progressing and, if anything, seemed to be getting better. However, her functional capacity was limited to class 3 of the scheme presented in chapter 2 (page 15). That's when she came to the Cooper Clinic for exercise therapy at our Cooper Fitness Center. I first met Cheryl in our medically supervised exercise program. As was true for her peers in the program, her still-fragile condition necessitated exercise under the watchful eyes of health professionals, ready to respond to any emergencies.

I started Cheryl on range-of-motion and stretching exercises plus isometric muscle-strengthening exercises like those that appear in chapter 3. After 4 weeks of isometrics, her strength had increased enough for her to start on isotonic exercises using resistance rubber bands, which she preferred to the hand-held weights that many of our other patients use. The rubber bands were easier for her to grip because her arthritis had caused finger deformities.

At the same time, Cheryl was doing an aerobic exercise program of stationary cycling and slow walking. I gradually increased the duration over 12 weeks until she was able to do 20 minutes of each

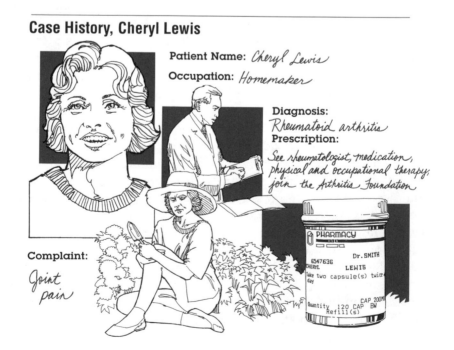

Case History, Cheryl Lewis

Patient Name: *Cheryl Lewis*

Occupation: *Homemaker*

Diagnosis:
Rheumatoid arthritis

Prescription:
See rheumatologist, medication, physical and occupational therapy, join the Arthritis Foundation

Complaint:
Joint pain

during a session. However, frequent fatigue made it necessary to introduce Cheryl to the concept of *interval training* (discussed in chapter 3, page 59). If aerobics made her unduly tired, she could slow down until she got a second wind—or, if really necessary, stop until she felt able to continue.

After 3 months in this program she was still earning less than 50 health points each week—the minimum recommended level (discussed in chapter 4). But her stamina and confidence were so much improved that I allowed her to go it alone from then on, *provided* she did only the exercises I assigned to her. If she wanted to branch out and try new physical activities, she had to confer with me first.

Today, Cheryl does water aerobics twice a week augmented with vigorous walks around the paths of our center. She fills in with stationary cycling and an occasional outdoor bike excursion with her family. It's the rare week when she earns 100 health points, but that's okay. For Cheryl, consistently earning over 50 points is all that I ask. Even that much is enough to confer the health benefits she needs to aid her recovery. The health benefits are already obvious: Her aerobic fitness has increased by almost 50% and her strength by a staggering 75%. Interval training is no longer necessary because her weakness and fatigue are substantially reduced. Although her medication hasn't changed since she's been exercising, she has less pain and stiffness overall in her joints.

I'm happy to report that the memory of her father's affliction no longer haunts Cheryl because it's clear to her that she's broken the mold. She's not confined to life in a rocking chair. Instead, she's actively pursuing the good life and is living proof that despite rheumatoid arthritis you can defy the odds. For Cheryl, the real bonus from her workouts is being able to garden again.

ARTHRITIS IN PROFILE

I've been using the term *arthritis* rather loosely. Strictly speaking, there are 127 different kinds of arthritis, some extremely rare, others quite common. Alan Hoffman and Cheryl Lewis represent the two most widespread forms, which I focus on in this book.

The word *arthritis* is derived from two Greek words. The first, *arthron*, means joint. The second, *itis*, means inflammation. Literally translated then, arthritis means *inflammation of a joint*. Those with only a cursory understanding of arthritis may mistakenly assume that inflammation is always a bad thing because it triggers arthritis pain.

Although inflammation is a sign of trouble, to be sure, it's actually a vital renewing process that occurs in response to injury of living tissue. It's a positive healing process *provided it ends in relatively short order and does not linger indefinitely and become chronic*. It's the chronic nature of arthritic inflammation that's negative and sets in motion the chain reaction leading to arthritic symptoms and signs (such as joint pain, tenderness, warmth, swelling, and redness) and complications.

Osteoarthritis has the distinction of being the oldest and most prevalent chronic disease known to humanity. It's a degenerative disease characterized by the progressive loss of joint cartilage (see Figure 1.1). Fortunately the damage is limited to the musculoskeletal system and it usually involves only one or a few joints. The weight-bearing joints—the feet, knees, hips, and spine—as well as the digital joints of the fingers, hands, and toes are most likely to be problem areas.

Until recently experts thought osteoarthritis resulted from normal wear and tear on a person's joints over the course of a lifetime. New studies, which compare the changes in an elderly person's joint cartilage with those in a younger person with osteoarthritis, make it clear that the cause is not that straightforward and unequivocal. These studies indicate that the two groups' conditions are not always identical. Thus, the current view is that a variety of factors interact to cause osteoarthritis.[3,4] These factors are aging, repetitive impact on the body's weight-bearing joints, genetics, and some other biochemical processes, as yet unknown.

In contrast, the characteristic feature of rheumatoid arthritis is inflammation of the synovial membranes that line the inside of certain joints (see Figure 1.1). Rheumatoid arthritis involves many joints and even moves beyond the musculoskeletal system to other areas of the body, making it challenging to treat. It's defined as "a chronic, multisystem, inflammatory disease whose cause is unknown." Rheumatoid arthritis's so-called "systemic complications," involving systems in the body other than the musculoskeletal system, are what make it so potentially devastating. But it is considerably rarer than osteoarthritis. Although rheumatoid arthritis is more likely to attack adults, especially women, middle-aged or older, it can occur in juveniles—and does.

AN OVERVIEW OF ARTHRITIS TREATMENT AND REHABILITATION

Today, those forward-thinking doctors (often family doctors) who treat arthritis patients know that full rehabilitation from this disease is a

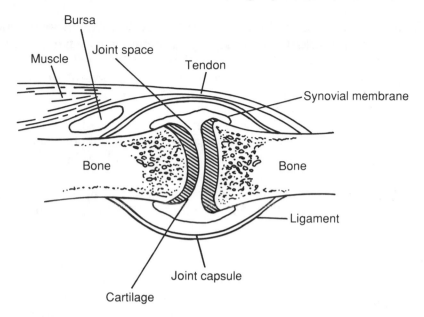

Figure 1.1   The components of a synovial joint. *Note.* From James F. Fries, *Arthritis,* © 1990, by Addison-Wesley Publishing Company, Inc. Reprinted with permission of the publisher.

DEFINITIONS

joint. The approximately 200 bones of the adult skeleton are attached to each other via connections called "joints." The most common and mobile joints in the body are synovial joints.

joint capsule. This tough, fibrous tissue completely surrounds the joint.

cartilage. The tough, pearly-blue, rubbery tissue that covers the ends of the bones in a synovial joint acts as a shock absorber, protecting the underlying bone.

synovial membrane. All surfaces within the joint capsule - with the exception of the cartilage - are lined by this thin "inner skin." It secretes synovial fluid into the joint space, making joint movement easy and smooth.

ligaments. These strong fibrous bands connect the ends of bones together.

tendons. These white, glistening, fibrous cords attach muscles to bones.

bursae. These fluid-filled sacs line various musculoskeletal surfaces that might otherwise experience too much friction as they rub against each other during joint movement.

daunting goal. Thus the best of them keep all their options open and delegate many tasks to better-equipped members of what could be termed an "arthritis rehabilitation team," an informal coalition of health-care specialists. Such a team comprises several of the following:[5]

- A rheumatologist (a specialist in the treatment of arthritis) or a physiatrist (a doctor who specializes in rehabilitation medicine)
- Nurses, such as those working in a rheumatology or orthopedic clinic
- Physical therapists (also known as physiotherapists), who use nonmedicinal methods for relieving pain and inflammation, including exercise; and exercise physiologists, who tailor exercise programs
- Occupational therapists, who work around physical disabilities to ease everyday life and enable patients to function independently
- Psychologists and medical social workers, who focus on the emotional, interpersonal, and financial issues that concern many severely disabled arthritis patients

At the center of all this expertise is the patient—you. You're the one person most responsible for reversing, or at the very least

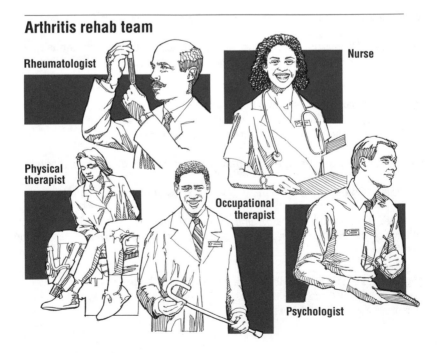

Arthritis rehab team

Rheumatologist

Nurse

Physical therapist

Occupational therapist

Psychologist

retarding, the course of your arthritis. None of these other specialists' counsel or the exercise rehabilitation advice in this book will do much good if you turn a deaf ear to it. When it comes to dealing with a chronic affliction like arthritis, *self-reliance* and *motivation* are important to keep in mind.

Chapter 2

Benefits and Risks of Exercise as an Arthritis Remedy

The Greek physician Hippocrates, in the fifth century B.C., first stated the principle implied in the popular dictum "Use it or lose it." Hippocrates wrote, "All parts of the body which have a function, if used in moderation and exercised in labours in which each is accustomed, become thereby healthy, well-developed and age more slowly. But if unused and left idle, they become liable to disease, defective in growth, and age quickly."[1]

Although this might strike contemporary readers as an astute observation, it was ignored for centuries. In fact, the medical community didn't give this notion much credence until the 20th century, choosing instead to champion rest therapy as the ideal and only way to treat arthritis and many other ailments. Even gentle exercise was considered harmful.

That's not what the experts are saying now. For several decades, doctors have been prescribing stretching ("flexibility") exercises because they help preserve joint function in people with arthritis, and indeed, in all aging people. Muscle-strengthening exercises are also recommended, provided they don't place too much stress on the joints. More recent evidence shows that regular aerobic exercise can also aid in arthritis rehabilitation. The Arthritis Foundation, among other authorities, currently approves range-of-motion, strength, and aerobic exercises, provided the exercise regimen is tailored for each patient and is coupled with appropriate rest.[2]

EXERCISE BENEFITS FOR THOSE WITH ARTHRITIS

It's useful to analyze an arthritis rehabilitation program in terms of its impact on "the four Ds"—death, disability, discomfort (psychological as well as physical), and dollar cost. In this chapter I'll discuss how a safe and inexpensive exercise program can, without causing orthopedic injuries or other medical complications, help you live longer and prevent arthritic disability and discomfort. Keep in mind that the following discussion, as well as the exercise programs and Health Points System in subsequent chapters, applies primarily to persons in classes 1 and 2 (and many in 3) of the functional capacity classification scheme shown in the box on page 15. However, most of it is unlikely to apply to those of you in class 4. Such individuals should not embark on the exercise programs I describe until their medical treatment and rehabilitation program has moved them into class 3 or lower.

Exercise Prevents Premature Death

If you pay attention to the latest health findings, you already know that an inactive lifestyle and low fitness, two traits that characterize many people with arthritis, increase a person's chances of developing several potentially fatal chronic diseases, including coronary artery disease, high blood pressure, diabetes, and possibly strokes and cancer.[3] As you may also know, coronary artery disease, which causes heart attacks, is the leading killer in the United States and most other industrialized nations. Though you may not necessarily die as a direct result of your arthritis, it can ease you into a lifestyle that's lethal. People who use their arthritis as an excuse to put their feet up and coddle themselves for the remainder of their days are likely to reduce the number of those days.

   In 1987, Dr. Kenneth E. Powell and his colleagues from the Centers for Disease Control in Atlanta scrutinized over 40 respected studies that began as early as 1950. The group's goal was to assess how, and

FUNCTIONAL CAPACITY
OF PEOPLE WITH ARTHRITIS

The American Rheumatism Association has devised the following functional capacity classification scheme to categorize people
according to the extent of the disability caused by rheumatoid
arthritis. This system is also applicable to persons with osteoarthritis and other forms of arthritis.

In chapter 5, I'll inform you of a more precise way to track
changes in your functional capacity over time. However, throughout this book I'll refer to the functional capacity classification
described here when providing you with exercise guidelines.

Class 1

Complete functional capacity with the ability to carry on all of
the usual duties of everyday life without handicaps.

Class 2

Functional capacity that's adequate to conduct normal everyday
activities despite the handicap of discomfort or limited mobility
of one or more joints.

Class 3

Functional capacity that limits people to performing few or none
of the duties of their usual occupation or self-care.

Class 4

People are largely or wholly incapacitated—they're bedridden or
use wheelchairs, permitting little or no self-care.

Note: Modified from "Therapeutic Criteria in Rheumatoid Arthritis" by O. Steinbrocker
et al., *Journal of the American Medical Association, 1949, 140*, pp. 659-662.
Copyright 1949, American Medical Association. Used by permission.

if, exercise can prevent deaths from heart disease.[4] They came to the
conclusion that physical inactivity is just as strong a risk factor for
premature heart disease death as the traditional risk factors we hear
so much about—cigarette smoking, high blood pressure, and a high

cholesterol level. Since the publication of Dr. Powell's overview, several more key studies have been completed, and they strongly support the Powell group's conclusions. One of these studies, our Aerobics Center Longitudinal Study, tracked more than 13,000 healthy male and female Cooper Clinic patients whose aerobic fitness varied from low to moderate to high.[5] The results of the 8-year follow-up of these 10,224 male and 3,124 female patients found that the death rates of the unfit soared compared with those with moderate and high fitness. Because the statistics were adjusted for age, a person's age was neutralized as a contributory factor in his or her death. The evidence is compelling that regular exercise can reduce the risk, by almost 50%, of dying from heart disease.[6]

How is this applicable to people with arthritis?

To date, no studies have specifically evaluated how exercise can alter, for good or ill, an arthritic person's risk of dying prematurely from heart disease. Yet when you consider that many of the elderly participants in the previously mentioned studies were undoubtedly suffering from osteoarthritis (because it's almost universal in people over 65 years old), a special study would hardly seem necessary. It seems logical to assume that people with osteoarthritis who exercise regularly will experience the same reduced risk of death from heart disease as active people without this condition. This seems all the more logical considering that there's no direct relationship between osteoarthritis, which is localized to the musculoskeletal system, and coronary artery disease, which involves the cardiovascular system.

Rheumatoid arthritis is another matter. Coronary artery disease is the leading cause of death in rheumatoid arthritis patients, just as it is in the general population.[7] Thus, it seems likely that regular exercise would prove effective in reducing the risk of premature death in anyone with this condition. However, rheumatoid arthritis does not confine its damage to the musculoskeletal system. In advanced cases, the skin, heart, lungs, nervous system, eyes, blood and blood vessels, spleen, and lymph nodes can be adversely affected. Some of these complications—referred to collectively as *systemic* complications be-cause they involve various organ systems throughout the body—can heighten a person's risk of dying prematurely. So the effect of regular exercise on the risk of dying from these systemic complications is still partly unknown.

Clearly, there's a wealth of investigating yet to be done in this area. One small-scale, 9-year study of 75 rheumatoid arthritis patients, conducted by Vanderbilt University School of Medicine researchers,

Systems affected by arthritis

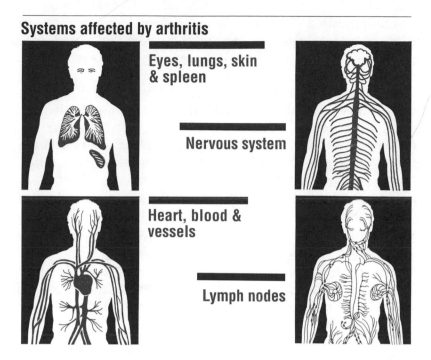

Eyes, lungs, skin
& spleen

Nervous system

Heart, blood &
vessels

Lymph nodes

sheds a little more light on the situation.[8] During the course of the study, 20 of the 75 subjects died. The causes of their deaths were similar to those for the general population, but the researchers were surprised by one particular finding: Low functional capacity tripled rheumatoid arthritis patients' risk of dying during the study period. Functional capacity was based on the subject's ability to (a) rise from a chair, walk 25 feet, and sit back down in a chair within a reasonable length of time and (b) undo and redo five buttons as quickly as possible. The researchers believe that the connection between low functional capacity and premature death "raises the possibility that aggressive therapy directed at improving functional capacity may be appropriate in rheumatoid arthritis." The obvious way to accomplish this is through a program of regular exercise.

Exercise Prevents Disability

Of all the chronic diseases, arthritis generally results in the most long-term disability. I believe this occurs, for one reason, because many physicians are still too cautious and conservative about their exercise prescriptions. Until recently the traditional exercise program for arthritis patients was built exclusively around range-of-motion exercises interspersed with lots of rest. When patients complained to their doctors about weakness and fatigue, they were told to reduce their amount of exercise even more, instead of being encouraged to increase it.

There's no doubt that appropriate rest helps reduce joint inflammation. However, it's also an established fact that excessive rest is deleterious to health.[9] Research shows that even in healthy young men only 3 weeks of lying prone in bed can reduce their fitness as much as 30 years of normal aging. In just 1 week of immobilization, a muscle can lose some 30% of its bulk!

The negative effects of immobility on the musculoskeletal system include these:

- Wasting (atrophy) of the muscles, tendons, ligaments, and bones
- Weakness of muscles, ligaments, tendons, and bones
- The development of contractures (a shortening or shrinkage of the muscles, tendons, ligaments, and joint capsules that reduces the range of a joint's motion and impairs mobility)
- Degeneration of joint cartilage
- Greater risk of breaking a bone due to the loss of bone mass, a condition called *osteoporosis*

Given these effects, it's somewhat paradoxical for physicians to answer their patients' complaints of fatigue, weakness, and disability with recommendations for more rest, which will further reduce their functional capacity—that is, their ability to perform occupational, recreational, household, and self-care activities. Such an approach sets in motion a vicious cycle of even more weakness, fatigue, loss of joint function, and disability. Today, enlightened exercise prescriptions for arthritis patients go beyond mere range-of-motion exercises and now often include muscle strengthening as well as aerobic exercise.

Why muscle strengthening? Muscle weakness is common in people with osteo- and rheumatoid arthritis—estimates are that 80% of all patients experience it.[10] You may think the disease of arthritis is the culprit. Yes, it's one cause. Another is *too little physical activity*. If you've been fairly active and then abruptly stop exercising, you'll find that the greatest decline in your strength occurs during the first days of your immobility. It continues thereafter, of course, but at a slower rate. If your immobility is total, as in the case of bed rest, your loss of strength may proceed at a rate of about 3% per day during the first week.[11]

Fortunately, studies show that arthritis patients can safely improve their strength, and thereby enhance their functional capacity, if they undertake an appropriate muscle-strengthening program.[12] A reasonable amount of strength is a prerequisite for performing many everyday activities. In other words, strength translates into good functional capacity and lessened disability. That's one of the reasons why it's important.

Why exercise aerobically? Aerobic exercises are endurance activities that don't require excessive speed or strength but do require demands on your cardiovascular system. There are many forms of aerobic exercise. Brisk walking, running, swimming, dancing, and cycling are perhaps the most popular, but there are others too. One objective of this type of exercise is to increase the maximum amount of oxygen that your body can process for energy production during physical activity. This enables you to perform more exercise with less fatigue.

There have been several major European and American aerobic exercise studies involving hundreds of people with osteo- and rheumatoid arthritis. Some of the studies lasted as long as 8 years. Dr. Robert W. Ike and his colleagues from the University of Michigan Medical Center reviewed the findings and came to these conclusions about typical osteo- and rheumatoid arthritis patients:[13]

- Their poor endurance and aerobic fitness levels are due as much to inactivity as to the disease. For many patients, traditional recommendations to reduce physical activity are inappropriate and may, in fact, contribute to their feelings of weakness and fatigue, as well as their impaired functional capacity.
- Such patients *can* perform aerobic exercise without harming their joints.
- These patients are often capable of substantially improving their aerobic fitness by participating in a supervised exercise program.
- Those who do participate in an aerobic exercise training program report improvements in many areas of functional capacity.

Exercise Relieves Physical and Psychological Discomfort

The main sources of physical discomfort for those with arthritis are joint stiffness and pain. There's documented proof that appropriate exercise can help alleviate both.

The majority of exercise studies using arthritis patients document an improvement, rather than a worsening, of their joint stiffness.

Researchers still don't know the precise reason for morning stiffness. One possibility is that the tissues surrounding the joint become water-logged during periods of inactivity. During rest, fluid leaks out of blood vessels into the joint tissues, making them feel stiff until joint motion begins to pump the fluid out of the tissues and back into blood vessels and lymph channels. If this theory is accurate, appropriate exercise could be expected to help rather than worsen the situation.[14]

One major complication of arthritis is the development of contractures, a shortening of muscles, tendons, ligaments, and joint capsules. Contractures make it very difficult, if not impossible, to extend or straighten out a joint completely. Contractures can develop within 1 week of inactivity, and because they're far easier to prevent than to correct, daily range-of-motion exercises are highly recommended. It's also important to keep joints extended—that is, fully straightened out—when you're sitting, standing, and, in particular, lying down. That means putting your feet up on a hassock or footstool in front of your easy chair, letting your arms droop at your sides when you're standing upright, and not bending your arms or legs when you're prone.

Pain, as you well know, is one of the toughest aspects of living with arthritis. Joint inflammation is the primary pain inducer for people

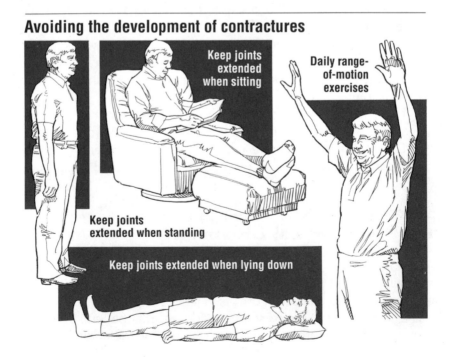

Avoiding the development of contractures

Keep joints extended when sitting

Daily range-of-motion exercises

Keep joints extended when standing

Keep joints extended when lying down

with rheumatoid arthritis. In people with osteoarthritis, inflammation is only one reason. Joint cartilage degeneration, which increases pressure on the joint bones, is another. Both arthritic conditions may also trigger painful muscle spasms, which are the muscles' attempt to splint and thus protect the joints from awkward movements.

When it comes to exercise and pain, I subscribe to the dictum that all competent doctors know to be true: *inappropriate physical activity worsens arthritis pain.* This is especially true if the arthritis in a joint is currently active. It's active if you experience noticeable inflammatory symptoms or signs such as joint swelling, warmth, redness, pain, and tenderness.

The key word here is *inappropriate*, not *exercise*. Many studies have shown that most people with osteo- and rheumatoid arthritis can derive the health-inducing benefits of exercise without aggravating their pain. Studies have shown that regular exercise helped lessen arthritis severity by reducing both the pain itself and the number of joints causing pain.[15-17]

The emotional pain triggered by knowing you have a chronic disease is often a far more daunting problem than mere physical pain. Arthritis forces many people to change their lifestyles and to worry, about the future in general and how to pay medical bills in particular.

Although I'd be foolish to claim that regular exercise is a panacea for psychological problems, I do know it can help profoundly, based on scientific as well as anecdotal evidence. Several studies have concluded that persons who are faithful exercisers suffer less from stress, anxiety, and depression; they sleep better and have an enhanced sense of self-esteem.[18] One participant in a 5-week Swedish aerobic exercise training study commented, "The physical training at the hospital was the best thing that has happened to me since I got rheumatoid arthritis 9 years ago."[19]

How does exercise affect self-esteem? It's well known in the exercise community that about half of all people who start an aerobics exercise program drop out within the first 6 months. If you can defy this statistic, imagine how you'll feel. In effect, exercise will come to symbolize your perseverance, your ability to make a commitment to something and stick with it through thick and thin. Exercise will provide tangible proof that you really do have more control than you thought over your condition. This knowledge will help prevent a syndrome known as *learned helplessness*, in which patients come to believe their affliction is totally beyond their control and must be borne with as much stoicism as possible. Learned helplessness results in a vicious downward spiral of further psychological problems and dependence on others. Taken to its logical conclusion, invalidism is the end result.

Ken Cooper likes to tout exercise as "nature's own tranquilizer." He and others believe that this tranquilizing effect occurs in part because aerobic exercise often triggers the release of endorphins, hormones produced by the pituitary gland in the brain. Once endorphins enter the bloodstream, their beneficial effects are thought to last several hours. Those effects are two-fold. The first is relief from pain, which may be one reason arthritic exercisers sometimes report a reduction in their usual joint aches; the second is a sense of euphoria, a feeling that all is right with the world.[20,21]

Exercise Provides Dollar Advantages

Arthritis is an expensive disease, not necessarily in terms of dollars expended for medical treatment, but in dollars lost when you're too disabled to work. In the United States musculoskeletal disorders, of all the disease groups, result in the most lost earnings. Each year the economic costs of musculoskeletal conditions approach 1% of our gross national product[22]—a staggering statistic! Half of all people ages 21 to 65 with rheumatoid arthritis are no longer capable of working 10 years after the onset of the disease.[23] Moreover, Americans sidelined with arthritis often find themselves forfeiting the generous health insurance benefits that only large-scale U.S. employers can afford to underwrite for their workers. Arthritis is ranked consistently among the leading medical diagnoses of people applying for social security disability benefits.

If exercise can improve a person's fitness and functional capacity, it can also enhance a person's productivity. Doesn't that translate directly into dollars earned?

I don't want to leave you with the impression that participating in an exercise program is free of expense. As an arthritis patient, you'll incur the cost of periodic medical evaluations and testing, fees for participating in a supervised exercise program or joining a health club, and payments for exercise equipment. Such expenses can be kept to a minimum. The first one—periodic medical checkups—is the only expense that the average exercising arthritis patient can't do without. But for those of you with less severe arthritis, the cost of a medical screening before you begin your program and the price of a good pair of walking shoes may be the extent of your financial outlay.

By now you should be convinced about the many benefits of a physically active lifestyle for persons with arthritis. However, please keep in mind that *exercise is not a panacea, but rather an extremely important supplemental therapy. To be most effective, regular exercise must be combined with appropriate medical care as well as other positive lifestyle changes* (correct nutrition, for example).

RISKS FROM EXERCISE

Yes, there are some exercise risks. The major health hazards of *vigorous* exercise for anyone, whether or not they have arthritis, are cardiac complications and musculoskeletal injuries. People with arthritis run the special risk of doing the wrong kind of exercise that could worsen their condition or any complications stemming from their condition.

Cardiac Complications

You've all read or heard about people who drop dead suddenly from a heart attack while exercising. It's a chilling picture that might make you wonder if it's safe to exercise, especially if you're up in years.

Studies make it clear that exercise itself is not the problem.[24] It's the lethal combination of injudicious, vigorous exertion and preexisting coronary artery disease that you may not know you have. In chapter 5 I'll tell you how to determine whether you might have coronary artery disease and, if you do, how to minimize your risk of a potentially fatal cardiac event during exercise. Be assured that when appropriate precautions are taken exercise is exceptionally safe even for most people with heart disease.

The same statement cannot necessarily be made about the various systemic complications of arthritis. To date, there have been few exercise-arthritis studies on patients with serious systemic complications involving the heart, lungs, nervous system, or blood vessels, so it's not possible to know exactly how safe exercise is for such patients. I suspect that some of these complications may be worsened by excessively vigorous exercise or predispose a patient to other exercise-induced problems. Thus anyone with a type of arthritis that is known to be associated with systemic complications must see his or her doctor before proceeding with our programs. Examples of such conditions include rheumatoid arthritis, systemic lupus erythematosus, systemic sclerosis, dermatomyositis, polymyositis, polymyalgia rheumatica, ankylosing spondylitis, Reiter's syndrome, psoriatic arthritis, Lyme disease, and arthritis associated with chronic inflammatory bowel disease.

Musculoskeletal Injuries

Even healthy adults who exercise occasionally suffer musculoskeletal injuries. Two recent studies estimate that some 50% of all competitive runners sustain at least 1 exercise-related injury each year.[25,26] However, these are serious amateur or professional runners. When the sample involves only recreational exercisers, the story is much different. Such studies, including one conducted at The Cooper Institute for Aerobics Research,[27] suggest that the number of exercise-induced injuries among noncompetitive athletes is not nearly as high as commonly believed. It's estimated that musculoskeletal injuries serious enough to require medical care probably occur at an annual rate of less than 5% among recreational exercisers. In chapter 5 I tell you how to take adequate precautions to minimize your risk for musculoskeletal injuries.

Some of you may still be skeptical about exercise and arthritis. Famous sports figures, such as Billie Jean King, have sustained repeated injuries and eventually developed osteoarthritis, usually after undergoing joint surgery. Exercise per se didn't cause their osteoarthritis. Repeated injuries and joint surgery did. Still, now that they have the disease, they, like you, need to know if high-impact activities such as running will worsen their condition. The answer is, "Yes, they could." I know many people with osteoarthritis who do run, but they use good judgment about it and take the necessary precautions. But I don't recommend running to persons with a moderate to severe case of osteoarthritis in their weight-bearing joints. The preferred activities for such individuals are low-impact aerobics such as walking, cycling, and swimming.

Chapter 2

Prescription

☐   Include exercise in your arthritis treatment/rehabilitation program.
☐   Exercise regularly to reduce your risk for premature death, minimize disability, relieve discomfort, and reduce the economic burden of your arthritis.

❐ Keep in mind that exercise is not a panacea, but rather an extremely important supplemental therapy.

❐ To gain optimal benefits, combine regular exercise with appropriate medical care and other positive lifestyle changes.

❐ Be aware that inappropriate exercise could worsen your arthritis and any complications stemming from it.

❐ Obtain your doctor's consent before embarking on an exercise program.

Chapter 3

Getting Started on a Regular Exercise Program

You could think of exercise as a form of arthritis "medication." When you exercise, just as when you take drugs, you have twin goals: *effectiveness* and *safety*. You must strike a balance between the two.

This chapter and the next will concentrate on effectiveness. I'll explain which types of exercise, and how much of each, you need to derive maximum health benefits. Chapter 5 will concentrate on safety. What constitutes safe exercise for an arthritis patient is quite different from safe exercise for a diabetes or cardiac patient, for example.

Even among arthritis patients, exercise regimens must be individually tailored to take into account the differences in the severities of their conditions. Although all the exercises depicted on these pages have been specifically designed for arthritis patients, I still urge you to check with your doctor before using them. Noticeable joint deformity or instability, previous joint surgery, or some other serious medical condition are reasons why you may have to avoid specific exercises—or not exercise at all for the time being.

THE COMPONENTS
OF AN EXERCISE WORKOUT

All exercise is not the same. For people with arthritis, the three most important types are

- range-of-motion and stretching (or flexibility) exercises,
- muscle-strengthening exercises, and
- aerobic exercise.

All three should be included ideally in a regular exercise program. Unfortunately, depending on your form of arthritis and the amount of pain and inflammation you have, this may not always be possible.

In a typical exercise session you should spend 10 to 20 minutes doing range-of-motion, stretching, and muscle-strengthening exercises. For the next 5 minutes do an aerobic warm-up, followed by 15 to 60 minutes of aerobic exercise at appropriate intensity. Spend 5 minutes cooling down aerobically, and finish your session with 5 minutes of range-of-motion and stretching exercises. You'll note that range-of-motion exercises, stretching, and strength-building (muscular conditioning) are done at the beginning; range-of-motion and stretching exercises are done again at the end of the workout. Please keep in mind that it may take you several weeks to work your way up to the durations I've specified for certain components.

Range-of-Motion and Stretching Exercises

Arthritis reduces a person's ability to move the joints through their full range of motion—one of arthritis's most devastating consequences. Impaired range of motion translates into a lower "functional capacity;" or a lessened ability to perform the usual activities of daily living—for example, bending down to retrieve something, combing your hair, or maintaining a garden.

It's now accepted that range-of-motion exercises are one important remedy for waning functional capacity. Range-of-motion exercises that employ a stretch at the end are especially helpful.

You may wonder why I recommend range-of-motion and stretching exercises both before and after a muscle-strengthening or aerobic workout. You open your exercise session with them primarily to limber up your body and reduce the chances of injury. When you do the exercises again after aerobics, you'll be surprised how much

Time spent in workout activities

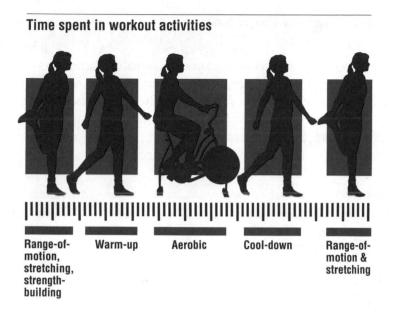

| Range-of-motion, stretching, strength-building | Warm-up | Aerobic | Cool-down | Range-of-motion & stretching |

easier they are. Why? Because your aerobic session has raised the temperature of the tissues surrounding your joints, making them more supple.[1]

A useful series of range-of-motion and stretching exercises are shown in Figures 3.1-3.12 and 3.13-3.17. By doing these exercises daily, you should gain some relief from stiffness, not to mention an improvement in flexibility.

You should never stretch or do any of these exercises to the point where they become painful or substantially worsen any pain that you had before the session. Use the arthritis pain scale described in chapter 5 (page 109); don't push yourself to where your rating of arthritis pain increases by more than 10 points during the session. If you experience a sudden, sharp pain, stop the exercise immediately. Also, check with your doctor before performing these exercises, particularly if you've had joint surgery or are in functional capacity class 3 (see box on page 15). Do not do these exercises if you are still in class 4.

There are other range-of-motion exercises and stretches beyond those detailed in this chapter. Should you wish to do others, I suggest that you do so only after discussing them with a health professional. Videotapes of an excellent exercise program called PACE (an acronym for "People with Arthritis Can Exercise") are available by contacting your local chapter of the Arthritis Foundation in the United States.

Range-of-Motion Exercises

For the 12 range-of-motion exercises described here, you'll be doing 3-5 repetitions of each, *provided* your pain rating is not above 70 on the arthritis pain scale (see page 109) and you have no other noticeable evidence of inflammation. With pain more severe than this or with other evidence of inflammation, limit yourself to 1 or 2 *gentle* repetitions of each. Keep in mind that joint range-of-motion exercises are meant to be done slowly with controlled movements.

Figure 3.1
Head Turns to Foster Neck Range of Motion.   Look straight ahead. Without raising or lowering your head, turn your head and look as far over your shoulder as possible. Hold that position for 2-3 seconds, and then return to your starting position. Repeat the same movement, this time looking over the other shoulder.

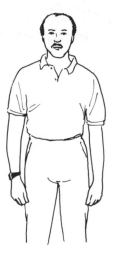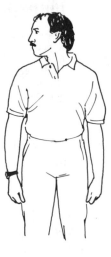

Figure 3.2
Head Tilt for Neck Range of Motion.   Keep looking straight ahead as you tilt your head so that your left ear moves toward your left shoulder. Hold that position for 2-3 seconds, and then return to your starting position. Repeat the same movement with the right ear and shoulder.

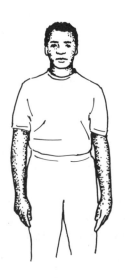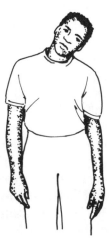

Figure 3.3
Arm Side-Raises for Shoulder Range of Motion.
Stand with your arms hanging at your
sides and your palms against the outside
of your thighs. Raise both arms sideways and up toward your ears, while
allowing your elbows to bend only
slightly. Hold that position for 2-3 seconds. Lower your arms to the starting
position and repeat.

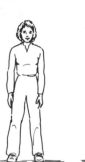
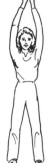

Figure 3.4
**Shoulder Front-to-Back Raises for Shoulder
Range of Motion.**   Stand with your arms
hanging at your sides and your palms
facing backwards. Raise your one arm
up in front of you towards the
ceiling, all the while keeping your
elbow as straight as possible. Simultaneously, raise your other arm up
behind you towards the ceiling,
likewise keeping your elbow as
straight as possible. Hold that
position for 2-3 seconds.
Lower your arms to the starting posi-
tion and repeat, alternating the arms you move forward and back.

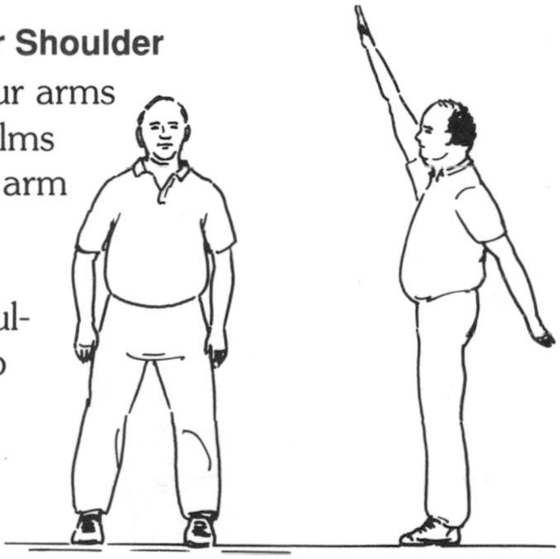

Figure 3.5
**Shoulder Blade Pulls for Shoulder
Blade Range of Motion.**   Bend
both elbows to a 90° angle. Lift
both elbows straight in front of
you and hold them at shoulder level,
your palms facing down and your
arms parallel to the floor. This is
your starting position. Keeping your
elbows bent, pull them sideways and
backwards, while trying to pinch
your shoulder blades together—
a position you should hold for
2-3 seconds. Return both elbows to the starting position and repeat.

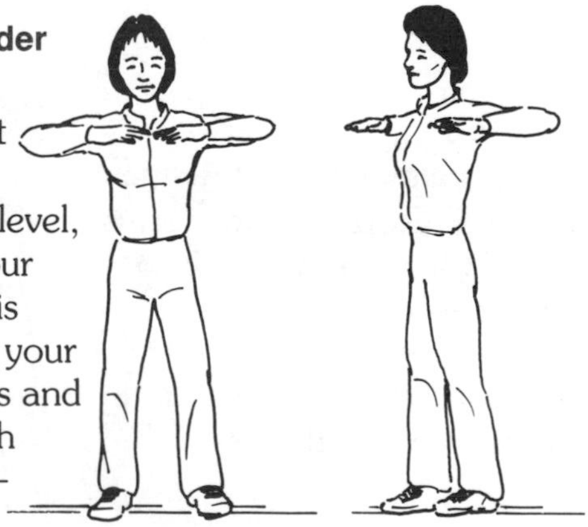

Figure 3.6
Side Bends for Back
Range of Motion.   Stand
with your arms hanging at
your sides and your palms
against the outside of your
thighs. Slide your one hand
down your thigh, keeping
your neck and back in a
straight line and without
leaning forward or backward.
Hold this position for 2-3
seconds. Return to the
starting position and
repeat with the other hand.

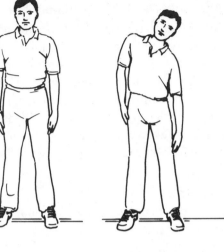

Figure 3.7
Elbow Curls for Elbow Range
of Motion.   Start with your
arms hanging at your sides
and your palms facing in
front of you. Keeping your
elbows close to your sides,
curl both hands up toward
your shoulders by bending
your elbows. Hold this
position for 2-3 seconds,
then lower your hands to the
starting position. Repeat.

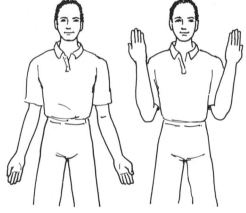

Figure 3.8
Wrist Circles for Wrist Range of
Motion.   Start with your arms
hanging at your sides. While
your arms remain stationary,
move your hands in a circle
in one direction and then in
the other. Repeat.

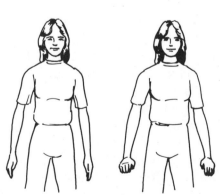

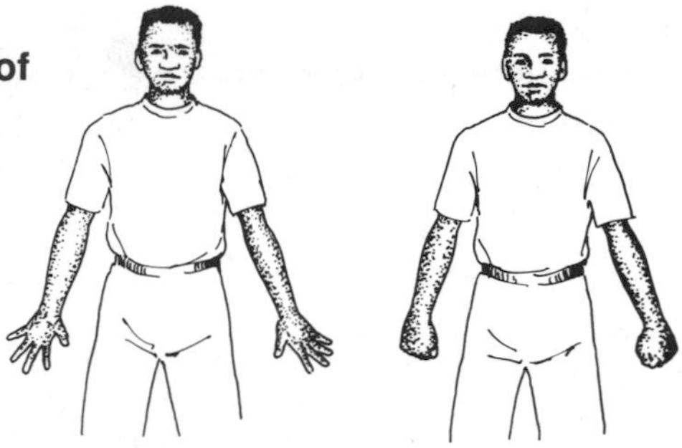

Figure 3.9
Finger Curls for Finger Range of
Motion.   Start with your arms
hanging at your sides and your
palms facing backward. Curl
all the fingers of both
hands—including your
thumbs—into a loose fist.
As you straighten your
fingers, spread them as far apart as possible. Repeat.

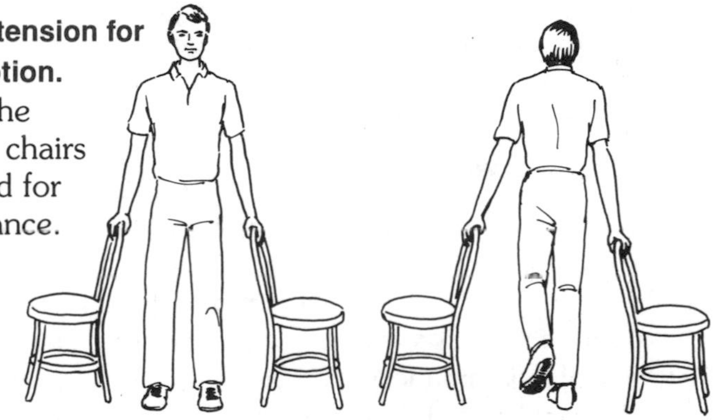

Figure 3.10
Standing Hip Extension for
Hip Range of Motion.
Stand between the
backrests of two chairs
that you can hold for
support and balance.
While keeping
your back as
straight as
possible, with
both knees
slightly bent and one foot in place, press the other leg as far backward as possible and lift it off the ground. Hold for 2-3 seconds.
Return the leg to the starting position and repeat with the other leg.

Figure 3.11
Supine Hip Abduction for
Hip Range of
Motion.   Lie flat on your
back with your legs extended on
the floor. Keeping one leg
straight in front of you,
slide the other leg as far
out to the side as pos-
sible. Hold for 2-3
seconds. Return the leg to
the starting position and repeat
the same action with the other leg.

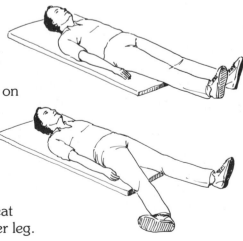

Figure 3.12
Ankle Circles for Ankle Range of Motion. Sit on the floor or on a chair and extend one leg out in front of you. While your leg remains stationary, move your foot in a circle in one direction and then in the other. Repeat with the other foot.

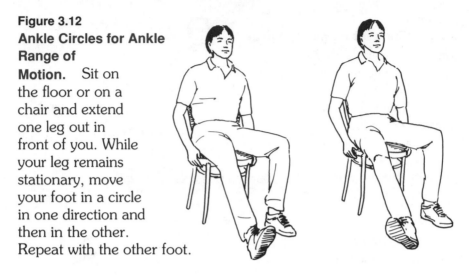

Stretching Exercises

Before and after each aerobic exercise session, do 1-3 repetitions of each stretching exercise shown here. Each stretch should be held for 10-20 seconds with no bouncing movements. If your pain is above 70 on the arthritis pain scale (see page 109), or you have other noticeable evidence of inflammation, limit yourself to 1 or 2 gentle repetitions of each. Remember to keep breathing—do not hold your breath.

Figure 3.13
Shoulder and Back Stretch. Lift your right elbow toward the ceiling and place your right hand as far down your back as possible between the shoulder blades. Allow your chin to rest on your chest. If possible, using your left hand, gently pull your right elbow to the left until a stretch is felt on the back of the right arm and down the right side of the back. Hold. Repeat with the left arm. If your arthritis pain is severe or accompanied by other signs of inflammation, do *not* use your hand to assist you in stretching.

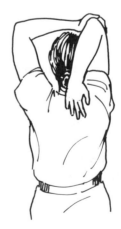

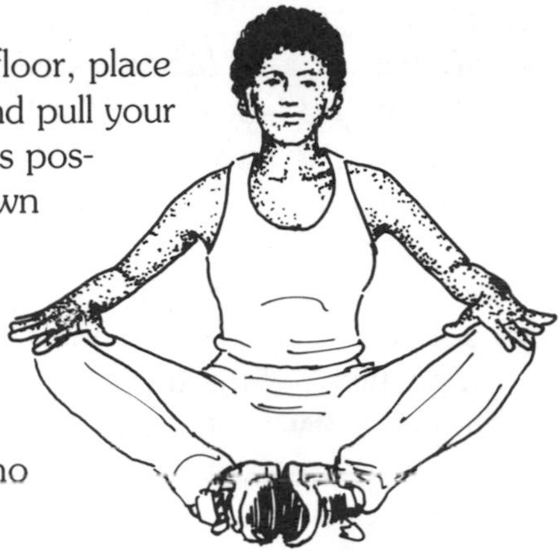

Figure 3.14

Inner Thigh Stretch.   Sit on the floor, place the soles of your feet together, and pull your heels in as close to the buttocks as possible. Gently press your knees down toward the floor. If your arthritis pain is severe or accompanied by other signs of inflammation, do not use your hands to help you do this stretch. This exercise should not be done by anyone who has had hip or knee surgery.

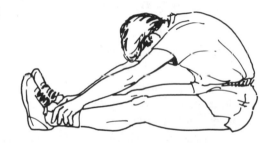

Figure 3.15

Lower Back and Hamstring Stretch.

Sit on the floor with your legs straight out in front of you and your hands on your thighs. Bend forward slowly, reaching toward your toes.

Keep your head and back aligned as you move into the stretch. If necessary, you can slightly bend your knees.

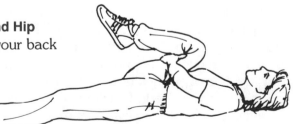

Figure 3.16

Lower Back, Thigh, and Hip Stretch.   Lie flat on your back with your legs extended on the floor. Pull your right knee up to your chest and press your back to the floor. Hold this position and then repeat with the left knee. If your arthritis pain is severe or accompanied by other signs of inflammation, do *not* use your hands to help you do this stretch. Don't do this exercise at all if you've had hip or knee surgery.

Figure 3.17
Calf Stretch.   Stand facing a wall, approximately 3 feet away. Place your palms on the wall, keeping your feet flat on the floor. Leave one foot in place as you step forward with the other. Make sure your back remains straight as you gently bend the front knee forward toward the wall. Repeat the same exercise with the opposite leg.

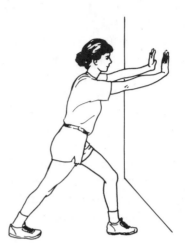

Muscle-Strengthening Exercises

Exercises to build muscle strength are also important for anyone with arthritis. I believe that both strength and flexibility are so important for optimal musculoskeletal health that, with funds from the National Institute of Arthritis and Musculoskeletal and Skin Diseases, I am conducting a 5-year study in this area that involves over 10,000 Cooper Clinic patients.

In contrast to flexibility training, which you can do daily and which you should include in all your workouts 3 to 5 days each week, muscle-strengthening exercises usually only need to be done 2 or 3 days a week—and *not* on consecutive days. Also, you may do your muscle-strengthening exercises after, rather than before, the aerobic portion of your workout. It's up to you.

The following series of isometric and isotonic strength-building routines—Figures 3.18-3.22 and 3.23-3.33, respectively—are easy enough for most arthritis patients to do at home with little risk of any adverse consequences. However, I still urge you to discuss this program with your doctor and get the okay to proceed. This is essential if you've had joint surgery, are in functional class 3 (see box on page 15), or currently have cardiovascular disease.

The workout series in Figures 3.18-3.22 shows *isometric* exercises. They're aimed at your muscles and involve the tensing of one set of muscles against another or against an immovable object—in this case, rubber bands. When you place the palms of your hands together and push, hold this position for several seconds, and then relax, you've just done an isometric exercise. It involves minimal or no joint movement.

The series in Figures 3.23-3.33 shows *isotonic* exercises. Like isometrics, isotonic exercises also require the contraction of muscles. But unlike isometrics they require the movement of a joint or limb. Weight lifting is a typical isotonic strengthening exercise.

Studies indicate that isometric exercises cause the least rise in pressure inside the joints, the least destruction of the bone ends that meet in the joints, and the least joint inflammation.[2] In addition, they've been shown to produce significant strength gains in people with arthritis.[3] Isometrics do have some drawbacks. For example, they don't develop strength throughout the full range of joint motion. In contrast, isotonics do and they generally result in greater strength gains according to a recent series of studies done at Tufts University in Boston.[4]

With a few exceptions, the following exercises use resistance rubber bands that are inexpensive (around $10), versatile, and convenient to use. Different types are available. "Dyna-Bands" and "Therabands," two of the most popular, can be ordered from The Hygenic Corporation, 1245 Home Avenue, Akron, OH 44310, telephone (216) 633-8460. This is how you exercise with them:

You either pull or push against the bands, which resist your efforts. The amount of resistance varies according to the thickness of the band you're using. The bands are color coded to indicate the thickness, thus the resistance. You can exercise with one band only or use them in combination for greater resistance.

Here are some exercise safety tips to bear in mind:

- Before you begin to exercise, make sure all jewelry, even a watch, is off your arms.
- For some of the exercises, you'll need to tie your band so it forms a loop. Use a knot or a half bow, which is easier to undo.
- During the exercise, always try to maintain the natural width of the band. Don't let it fold over.
- Maintain good posture throughout the exercise sequence.
- A Valsalva maneuver is exhaling forcefully without actually releasing air from the lungs. Doing this during an exercise is ill-advised.
- Never hold your breath during repetitions either. If you feel inclined to do so, it could be a sign that the band offers too much resistance for your current strength level. This is forcing you to strain when you shouldn't have to. Try counting out loud to make sure you're breathing normally.
- Start slowly and progress gradually. If you're weak to start with— as many of you in functional capacity class 3 (see box on page 15) will probably be—it won't take much exercise to improve your

strength. According to the results of one study, such people can increase dramatically their strength just by performing our isotonic exercise program working against gravity and without adding any resistance or weight at all.[5] When using the bands for isotonic exercises, start with the thinner ones and only progress to thicker ones if you can tolerate them. Keep in mind that increased resistance places greater stress on your arthritic joints.

If you have arthritis only in one or two joints—and you are in functional capacity class 1 or 2 (see box on page 15)—your doctor may not only encourage you to go ahead with our strength-building exercise program but may clear you to progress from ours to an even more strenuous one. If so, I encourage you to find an adequately trained health professional who is familiar with your case and willing to instruct you in the correct use of resistance-training equipment. A well-equipped gym might be outfitted with weight-training devices carrying such brand names as Cybex Strength Systems, Hydrafitness, Nautilus, and Universal. These are excellent machines provided someone carefully instructs you how to use them and supervises your exercise, at least initially. I also suggest you read *The Strength Connection*, which gives more detailed information on strength training.[6]

The American College of Sports Medicine recommends that the average healthy adult perform at least 2 times a week a minimum of 8 to 10 strengthening exercises involving the major muscle groups. They further urge adults to perform at least one set, consisting of 8 to 12 repetitions, of each strength-building exercise during each muscle-strengthening workout. If your doctor has cleared you to undertake a serious strength-training program, these recommendations may also be appropriate for you.[7]

Isometric Muscle-Strengthening Exercises Using Resistance Rubber Bands

Isometric exercises are of particular value for painful or inflamed joints. Use these exercises in preference to isotonic ones for joints that are moderately painful (rating of 30 or above on the scale on page 109) or with other noticeable inflammatory signs. If you are in functional capacity class 3 (see box on page 15), use isometric strengthening exercises before progressing to isotonic ones. Here are specific pointers for the following 5 isometric exercises:

- Do 1-3 repetitions daily of each of the following 5 exercises.

- Use the thickest band, which provides the most resistance and affords the least joint movement.
- Do only 1 repetition of each exercise if you have a pain rating above 70 (see page 109), or if you have pain accompanied by noticeable inflammation. If your pain is between 30 and 70 on the scale with no noteworthy inflammation, aim for 3 repetitions.
- During each repetition, push or pull as hard as you can for 6 seconds. Rest for 15-20 seconds between each repetition. Between each exercise, rest 15-60 seconds.
- Never hold the muscle contraction for more than 6 seconds because this could cause an excessive rise in blood pressure.

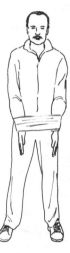

Figure 3.18

Shoulder Press (shoulders and, to a lesser degree, the upper back).   Place a looped band around your forearms, just above your wrists. Stand with your arms hanging in front of you, elbows slightly bent, and your palms facing each other. Keeping your elbows slightly bent, try to push your arms outward as hard as possible and maintain the effort for 6 seconds. The band resistance should be such that your arms move only a few inches apart or not at all. Relax and either repeat or go on to the next exercise.

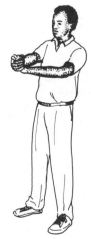

Figure 3.19

Chest Press (chest muscles and, to some extent, the upper back).   No bands are required for this exercise. Clasp your hands and extend your arms out in front of you at chest height. Keeping your elbows slightly bent, press the palms of your hands against each other as hard as you can and maintain the effort for 6 seconds. Relax and either repeat or go to the next exercise.

Figure 3.20
Combined Biceps Curl and Triceps Extension (biceps [or muscles in the front of the upper arm] and the triceps [or muscles in the back of the upper arm]). Place a looped band around your forearms, just above your wrists. Hold both arms gently against the front of your upper body, with your elbows bent at about a 90° angle and one forearm just above the other. Turn the palm of the top hand so that it's facing upwards and the palm of the bottom hand so that it's facing downwards. For 6 seconds, try as hard as you can to bend your top elbow and straighten out your bottom elbow, all the while keeping your forearms against your body and without changing your palms' direction. The band's resistance should be such that as little elbow movement as possible takes place. Relax and repeat the exercise, exchanging arm positions.

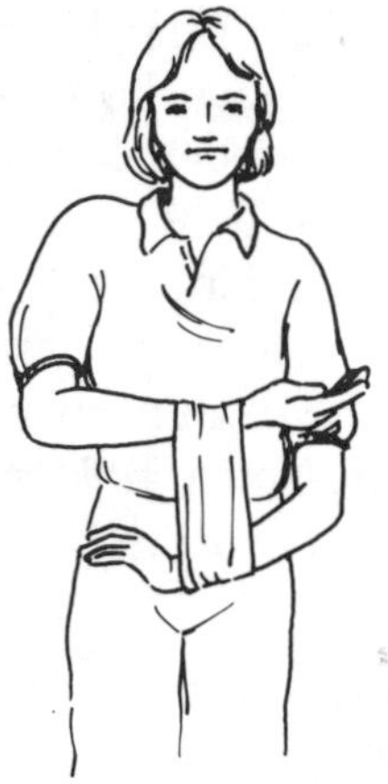

Figure 3.21
Standing Hip Flexion (hips, front of the thighs, and, to a lesser degree, abdominal muscles).   Stand between the backrests of two chairs with your feet close together. Place a looped band around the outside of your ankles. Throughout this exercise, hold onto both backrests for balance and support and keep both knees slightly bent. Bracing yourself with your arms and keeping one foot in place, press the other leg forward as hard as possible. The band's resistance should be such that your leg moves only a few inches forward or not at all. Maintain this stance for 6 seconds. Return your leg to your starting position and repeat with the opposite leg.

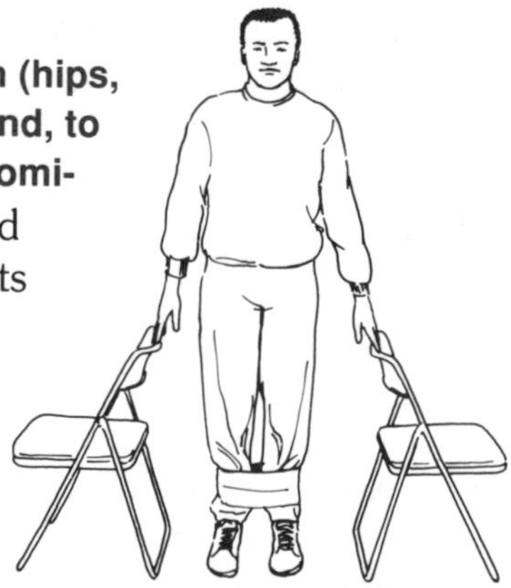

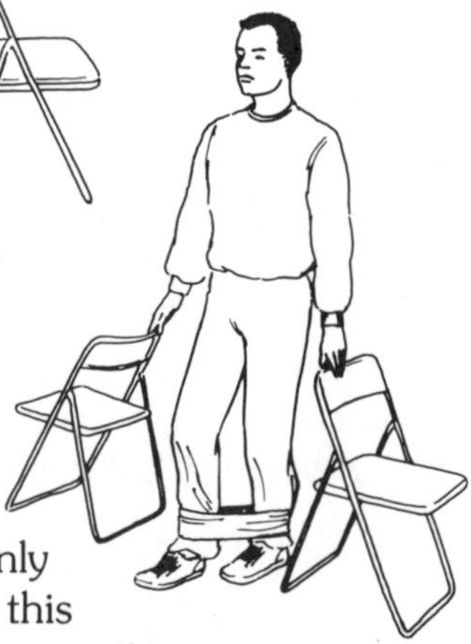

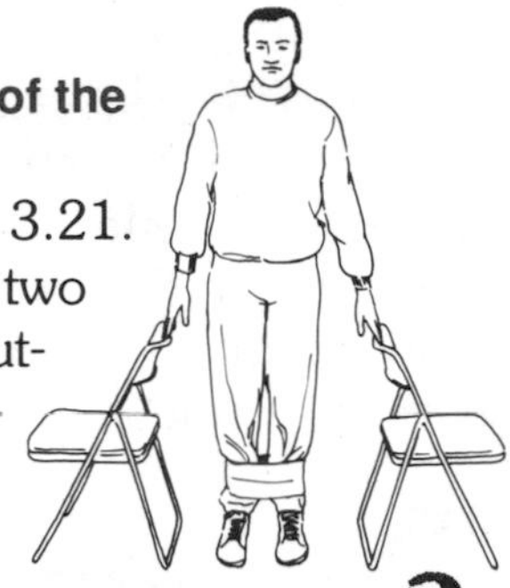

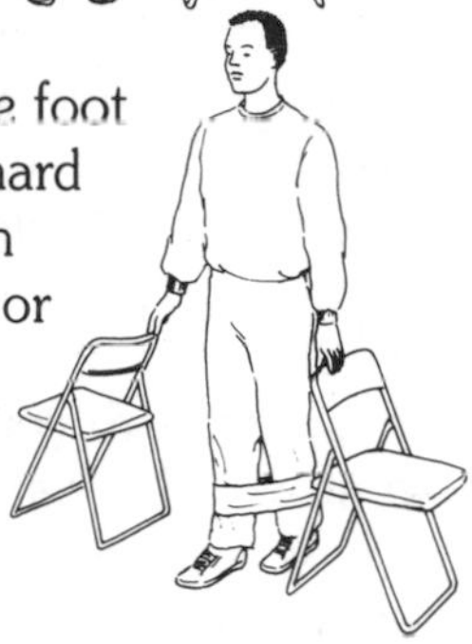

Figure 3.22
Standing Hip Extension (the hips, back of the thighs, buttocks, and lower back muscles). This is a variation of Figure 3.21. Once again, you'll be standing between two chairs with a looped band around the outside of your ankles. Hold onto the backrests of both chairs for balance and support and keep your knees slightly bent as you move through this exercise. Bracing yourself with your arms and keeping one foot in place, try to press the other leg backward as hard as possible. The band's resistance should be such that your leg moves only a few inches backward or not at all. Maintain this stance for 6 seconds. Return your leg to your starting position and repeat with the opposite leg.

Isotonic Muscle-Strengthening Exercises Using Resistance Rubber Bands

I recommend that you do these exercises 3 days a week on alternate days, following these guidelines:

- If you have arthritis in your hands or fingers, it may be a challenge to keep the band from slipping out of your grip. If so, you may need to tie loops at each end and attach them around your hands or wrists. This will necessitate ordering bands longer than the standard 36 inches (91 cm).
- When wrapping a band around any part of your body, do it so that you're still comfortable. It should never be too tight.
- Begin exercising with the thinnest band, which provides the least resistance. As your tolerance permits, gradually progress to the thicker bands.
- For each exercise, do 8-16 slow, complete, and controlled repetitions. Each execution should take from 3-5 seconds and your movements should be smooth and continuous. Never jerk your band or allow it to snap back. Always keep some tension on the band as it returns to its starting position, when you can relax completely for 2-3 seconds between repetitions. You control the band. Don't let it control you.

• Take 15-60 seconds to rest between each exercise. (The full number of repetitions ordered for each exercise is a *set*.) Once you've reached the point where, with relative ease, you can do 2 complete sets—2 × 16 repetitions for each exercise—you may want to progress to a thicker, more resistant band. However, keep in mind that it's far more important to do the exercises correctly than to increase the amount of resistance.

Figure 3.23
Side Shoulder Raise (outer portion of the shoulders).
Place your foot on one end of the band and grip the other end with the hand on the opposite side of your body. Start with your arm extended at your side and the palm of your hand facing the side of your thigh. Keeping your elbow slightly bent, raise your arm out at your side

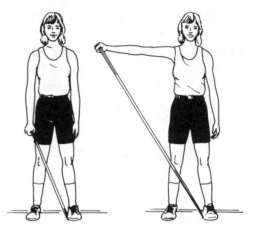

to shoulder level. Slowly lower your arm to the starting position. Repeat this motion with the same arm until you fulfill your repetition goal. Then switch to the other arm and leg and repeat.

Figure 3.24
Front Shoulder Raise (front portion of the shoulders).   This is a variation of Figure 3.23. Once again, place your foot on one end of the band, but this time grip the other end with the hand on the same side of your body. Begin with your arm extended at your side and the palm of your hand facing the side of your thigh. Keeping your elbow slightly bent, raise your arm out in front of your body to shoulder level.

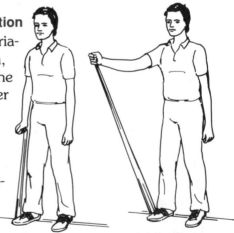

Slowly lower your arm to the starting position. Repeat this motion with the same arm until you fulfill your repetition goal. Then switch to the other arm and leg and repeat.

Figure 3.25
Chest Press (chest muscles and upper back). Loop the band around your upper back and grip the ends in your hands. Bend both elbows to a 90° angle. Lift both elbows away from your sides until they're at armpit level and your arms are almost parallel to the floor. This is your starting position. Press your arms forward until they're almost completely straight. Slowly bend your elbows until your hands return to the starting position. Repeat.

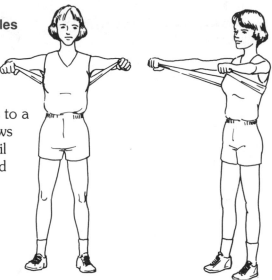

Figure 3.26
Biceps Curl (muscles in the front of the upper arm). Place your foot on one end of the band and grip the other end with the hand on the same side of your body. Start with your arm extended at your side and the palm of your hand facing forward. Keeping your elbow close to your side, bend it so that your fist curls upward to your shoulder. Slowly lower your arm to the starting position. Repeat this motion with the same arm until you fulfill your repetition goal. Then switch to the other arm and leg and repeat.

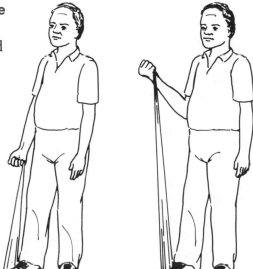

Figure 3.27
**Triceps Extension (muscles in the
back of the upper arm).** Take
one step forward and place your
front foot on one end of the
band. Grip the other end with the
hand on the *opposite side* of
your body. Bend your front
knee slightly, lean forward,
and rest the hand on the
same side of the body,
palm down, on your knee.
Place the other hand—the
one holding the band—against your hip,
palm facing inward. Gradually straighten
that arm out fully behind you. Then slowly
bend your arm until your hand returns to the
starting position at your hip. Repeat this
motion with the same arm until you fulfill your
repetition goal. Then switch to the opposite
arm and leg and repeat.

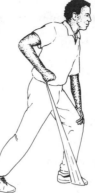
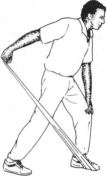

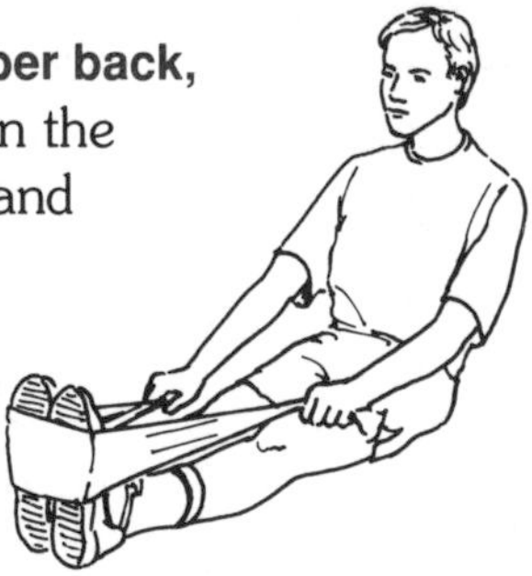

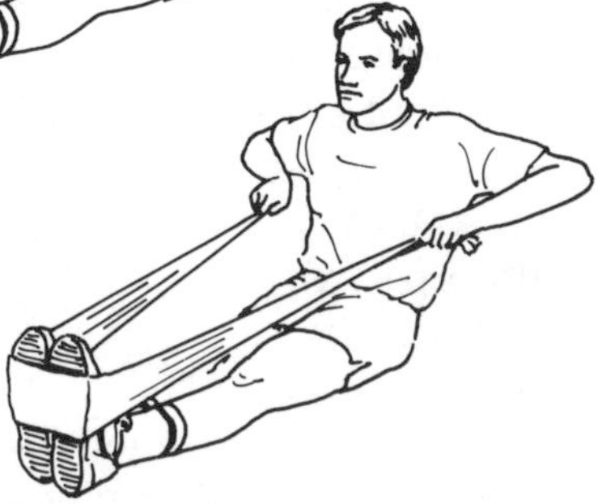

Figure 3.28
**Seated Rowing Exercise (upper back,
shoulders, and neck).** Sit on the
floor with your back upright and
your knees either bent or
straight, whichever is more
comfortable. Grab each
end of the band with
your hands and loop the
band around your feet.
Start with your arms ex-
tended in front of you, your hands
slightly lower than shoulder level,
and your palms facing the floor.
Pull both ends of the band toward
your armpits, while maintaining
good posture. Slowly return your
hands to the starting position and repeat.

Figure 3.29
Seated Hip Abduction (hips and outer thighs).   Sit on the floor with your back upright and your legs out straight in front of you. Place a knotted band around the outside of your ankles. Keep your legs straight as you brace yourself with palms on 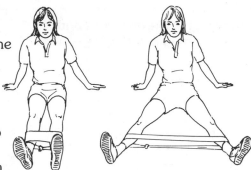 the floor just behind you. Slide your legs apart until you note significant resistance. Slowly return both legs to the starting position and repeat. To decrease the resistance, do this exercise with the band looped around the outside of your thighs just above the knees.

Figure 3.30
Half-Situps (abdominal muscles). Lie on the floor with your knees bent at a 90° angle and the palms of your hands resting on the front of your thighs. Lift your shoulders off the floor and slide your fingers up toward your knees. Return to the horizon- 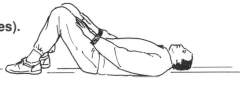 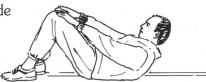 tal starting position and repeat.

Figure 3.31
Calf Raises (calf muscles).   Stand with your fingers against a wall in front of you for balance. Rise up onto the balls of both feet. Lower your heels to the floor and repeat. Keep your knees straight throughout this exercise.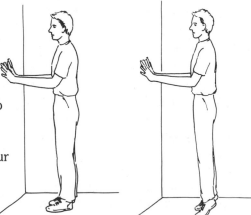

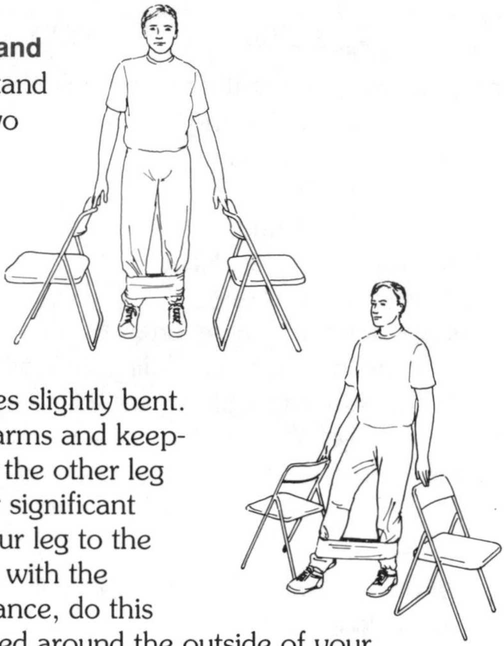

Figure 3.32
Standing Hip Flexion (hips and the front of the thighs). Stand between the backrests of two chairs with your feet close together. Place a looped band around the outside of your ankles. Throughout this exercise, hold onto both backrests for balance and support and keep both knees slightly bent. Bracing yourself with your arms and keeping one foot in place, press the other leg forward until you encounter significant resistance. Slowly return your leg to the starting position and repeat with the opposite leg. For less resistance, do this exercise with the band looped around the outside of your thighs just above the knees.

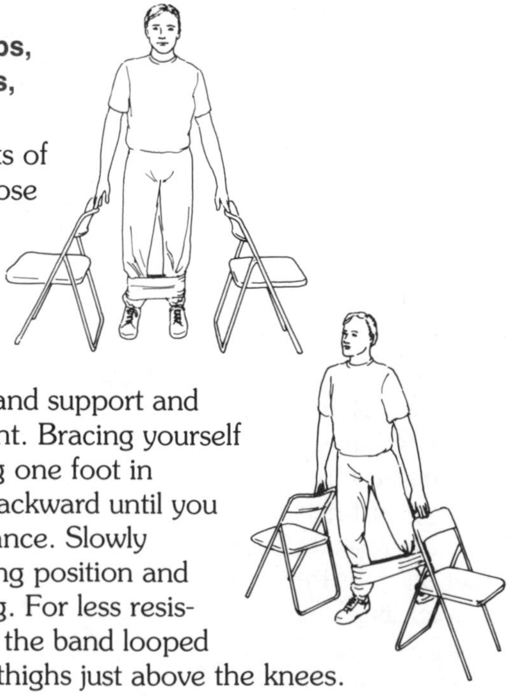

Figure 3.33
Standing Hip Extension (hips, back of the thighs, buttocks, and lower back muscles). Stand between the backrests of two chairs with your feet close together. Place a looped band around the outside of your ankles. Throughout this exercise hold onto both backrests for balance and support and keep both knees slightly bent. Bracing yourself with your arms and keeping one foot in place, press the other leg backward until you encounter significant resistance. Slowly return your leg to the starting position and repeat with the opposite leg. For less resistance, do this exercise with the band looped around the outside of your thighs just above the knees.

Aerobic Exercise

Ken Cooper coined the term *aerobics* in 1968 when his first book, *Aerobics*, was published.[8] Before Ken's influence, the dictionary defined *aerobic* as an adjective meaning "growing in air or in oxygen." It was commonly used to describe bacteria that need oxygen to live. Ken, however, used the word *aerobics* as a noun to denote those forms of endurance exercises that require increased amounts of oxygen for prolonged periods of time. The 1986 edition of the Oxford English Dictionary now defines *aerobics* as "a method of physical exercise for producing beneficial changes in the respiratory and circulatory systems by activities which require only a modest increase of oxygen intake and so can be maintained."

This is the key question you need answered: How much aerobic exercise is enough to insure health benefits without significantly increasing my risk of injury or aggravating my condition?

Dr. Steven N. Blair, Director of Epidemiology at The Cooper Institute for Aerobics Research, and other researchers from prestigious medical institutions in the United States have tackled this issue in depth.[9-11] Their answer is embodied in our Health Points System. They reviewed the findings of many exercise research studies and were able to identify an ideal upper and lower limit of exercise. Though future research studies are needed to clarify fully the situation, there appears to be a just-right level of exercise. This is actually a modest amount, nothing like the extremely strenuous workouts that exercise enthusiasts engage in as a matter of course. In the language of exercise physiologists,

> exercise training that results in a weekly energy expenditure between *10 and 20 calories per kilogram of body weight** is likely to bring about the major health benefits.[9] Twenty calories is the upper limit necessary from a health promotion standpoint— energy expenditures above this level do not appear to provide substantially more benefit. The lower limit of 10 calories is necessary to insure effectiveness,[10] although lesser amounts are still likely to be of some benefit.[12]

Here are two examples: Alan Hoffman weighed 220 pounds (or 100 kilograms) when he first arrived at The Cooper Aerobics Center. Therefore, he needed to work toward expending 1000 (or 100 × 10) to 2000 (or 100 × 20) calories during exercise each week. In contrast, Cheryl Lewis weighed 132 pounds (or 60 kilograms). Her target weekly

---

*1 kilogram (kg) = approximately 2.2 pounds. 1 calorie = approximately 4.2 kilojoules.

energy expenditure during exercise was 600 (or 60 × 10) to 1200 (or 60 × 20) calories.

These conclusions form the mathematical basis of the Health Points System you will encounter in the next chapter. Our Health Points System transforms these energy expenditure recommendations into a practical, easy to follow method of assessing the effectiveness of your exercise program. So if you're concerned about the complexity of calculating your weekly energy expenditure, you can stop worrying—our Health Points System will take care of this for you. Without it, most arthritis patients have no way of knowing how much exercise is needed to expend 10 to 20 calories per kilogram of body weight.

Factors That Determine Energy Expenditure

Weekly energy expenditure during exercise depends largely on four factors: the *type, frequency, intensity,* and *duration* of your exercise sessions. Your health-care team's job is to tailor a safe weekly exercise regimen for you using these four factors. Keeping both your medical condition and personal preferences in mind, your health-care team must help you

- choose a suitable aerobic exercise,
- decide on the number of times you should work out each week,
- determine the appropriate intensity at which to perform exercise, and
- establish how long each exercise session should last.

Before I tackle the issue of which aerobic exercise is right for you, you need to understand how the last three concepts intertwine. They're embodied in the concept of FIT, which is an acronym for **F**requency, **I**ntensity, and **T**ime. *Frequency* refers to *how often* you exercise. *Intensity* refers to *how hard* you exert yourself. *Time* refers to each exercise session's *duration*. An equation showing their interrelationship would look like this:

$$\text{Frequency} + \text{Intensity} + \text{Time} = \text{Caloric Energy Expenditure}$$
$$= \text{Health Benefit}$$

If the right side of the equation—that is, caloric energy expenditure and health benefit—is to remain constant but you cut down on one or two elements on the left side of the equation, the third element on the left side must increase to make up the difference. For example, if you exercise at a low-to-moderate intensity 3 days a week, each exercise session may have to last a relatively long time if you're to get enough exercise to have a substantial impact on your health. So if you exercise at that intensity but for a shorter length of time each session, you must increase the number of times per week you exercise to achieve the desired weekly energy expenditure.

Here are my recommendations concerning each of these factors:

Frequency.   I recommend 3 to 5 days per week as the ideal exercise schedule for people with and without arthritis. Less frequency of exercise is unlikely to produce significant health improvements; more predisposes you to musculoskeletal injuries and may even worsen some people's arthritis. You should space your workouts throughout the week. For example, if you're a 3-day-a-week exerciser, rather than training on Monday, Tuesday, and Wednesday, schedule your workouts for Monday, Wednesday, and Friday.

Time or Duration.   The higher the intensity or frequency, the shorter the time needed to attain the desired weekly energy expenditure. For arthritis patients, moderate-intensity aerobic exercise of longer duration is preferable to high-intensity exercise of shorter duration, for these reasons: (a) It lessens the risk of training-related complications, (b) it is less stressful on your musculoskeletal system, and (c) the average person is more likely to enjoy more moderate workouts. Longer, moderate workouts are particularly important if weight loss is a goal, because they promote fat loss while reducing the risk of musculoskeletal injuries.

Workouts of 30 to 45 minutes are ideal for most people with arthritis, but pain is sometimes a problem. Preliminary research conducted at Stanford University offers an alternative: Three 10-minute exercise sessions spread throughout the day may result in fitness gains similar to one 30-minute session.[13] This finding should be welcome news to all arthritis patients who find that shorter exercise sessions cause them less arthritis pain.

Bear in mind that the recommendations regarding duration do not include the warm-up and cool-down periods that should open and close each aerobics session. Take at least 5 minutes to ease into aerobics, starting at low intensity and slowly building up to your peak, target intensity. You should also reduce gradually your exercise intensity for 5 minutes at the end of your workout.

Intensity.   It's a fallacy to assume that you must exercise at a high intensity to derive health-related benefits. In short, the "no pain, no gain" axiom is wrong and is especially dangerous for people with arthritis. High-intensity exercise is more stressful to your joints than

Fitness gains through intermittent exercise sessions

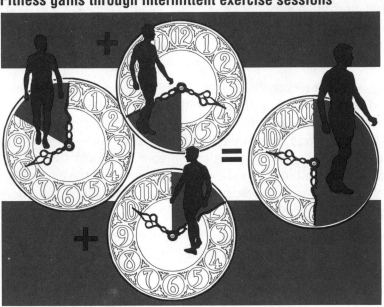

lower-intensity exercise, and it places people with cardiovascular problems at greater risk for exercise-related complications, including sudden death. Fortunately, it is now known that you can obtain optimal health-related benefits with a minimum of risk when you exercise at a moderate rather than a high intensity.

How to Quantify Exercise Intensity

There are a number of ways to quantify exercise intensity. I'll discuss 3 that you can choose from: METs, your heart rate, or your perceived exertion.

METs. The acronym MET stands for "metabolic equivalent unit." One MET is the amount of oxygen your body consumes for energy production each minute while you're at rest. If you're engaged in an activity corresponding to 5 METs, this means that your body is now taking up and using 5 times more oxygen than it did at rest. This is the amount your body now needs to fuel your working muscles, enabling them to produce the required amount of energy. (I'll return to the subject of METs later in this chapter when I discuss how to select an appropriate speed or work rate for the initial weeks of a walking or stationary cycling exercise program.)

Heart Rate. This is perhaps the most widely used and helpful way to target exercise intensity. This method is based on the principle that there's a direct relationship between the increase in your body's oxygen uptake during exertion and the increase in your heart rate.

I advise patients with arthritis to exercise at an intensity that raises the heart rate above 60% of their maximal heart rate but definitely no higher than 85%. That's an exercise training zone range spanning 25 percentage points. I have found that an exercise heart rate in the range of 60% to 75% of the maximal heart rate is ideal for most arthritis patients.

What's your maximal heart rate? The figure varies depending on the individual. Your maximal heart rate is the highest rate *you* are capable of attaining during exercise without experiencing musculoskeletal pain of sufficient magnitude to warrant stopping, and without developing significant cardiac abnormalities.

The most accurate way to determine your maximal heart rate is to take a treadmill or cycle exercise test. In medical jargon, it's called a "symptom-limited maximal exercise test with electrocardiogram (ECG) and blood pressure monitoring." (The term "symptom-limited" means that you continue exercising until you cannot go any further or until you develop certain ECG or other abnormalities that are an indication for your physician to stop your test.) I strongly advocate such a test for all our arthritis patients and encourage you to have one.

Both Alan Hoffman and Cheryl Lewis had exercise tests. Alan's maximal heart rate was 162 beats per minute. Cheryl's was 164 beats per minute.

Without a test, you'll have to use one of the following formulas to *estimate* your maximal heart rate:

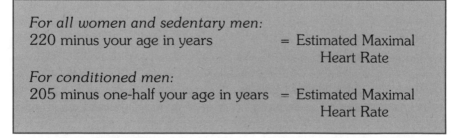

For all women and sedentary men:
220 minus your age in years .... = Estimated Maximal Heart Rate

For conditioned men:
205 minus one-half your age in years = Estimated Maximal Heart Rate

For example, Alan Hoffman at age 52 had an estimated maximal heart rate of 168 beats per minute (220 − 52 = 168) before starting our supervised exercise program; had he already been engaged in an exercise program, it would have been 179 beats per minute (205 – 26 = 179). At age 46, Cheryl Lewis' estimated maximal heart rate was 174 beats per minute (220 – 46 = 174). Note that Alan's actual maximal heart rate was 162, slightly lower than his estimate. Cheryl's was also lower; her actual value was 164.

But please be aware that these formulas are invalid for people taking medications—such as beta-blockers— that slow down the heart rate. For safety reasons, I also caution people who know they have heart disease to ignore these formulas, whether or not they're taking medication. In the place of these formulas, people in these categories should have their maximal heart rate determined by performing an exercise test. They should also be sure to use the Borg Perceived Exertion scale I'll describe later.

Training Target Heart Rate Zone.   Once you know your maximal heart rate (estimated from the formulas given, or precise, based on your performance during an exercise test) it's easy enough to determine the parameters you should stay within when you exercise. I recommend that you push your heart rate above 60% of your maximal heart rate but go no higher than 75%—and absolutely no higher than 85%. This is your *training target heart rate zone*, which you calculate by multiplying your maximal heart rate by the lower limit of 60% (.6) and the upper limit of 75% (.75).

Using Alan's actual maximal heart rate of 162, he calculated a lower limit of 97 beats per minute (or 162 × .6 = 97) and an upper limit of 122 beats per minute (162 × .75 = 122). Cheryl's training target heart rate zone was between 98 (164 × .6 = 98) and 123 (164 × .75 = 123) beats per minute.

This zone is important. Studies show that exercise performed at an intensity lower than 60% may net some health benefits but is unlikely to increase substantially your level of fitness.[14,15] Moreover, in lieu of exceeding the 60% mark, you'll probably have to lengthen your exercise sessions to well over an hour each time to attain the weekly energy expenditure I recommend. On the other hand, if you're under time pressure and can only work out a maximum of 3 days a week or for short durations, you'll be forced to exercise near the upper limit of your training target heart rate zone to gain any appreciable health benefit.

Keep in mind that it's crucial never to exceed the 85% upper limit; the only exceptions are for competitive athletes. Why? Because during such high-intensity exercise, you are placing unnecessary stress on your musculoskeletal system. For people with cardiovascular problems, intensities above the 85% limit also increase their risk for triggering a cardiac complication during exercise.

Using Heart Rate to Guide Intensity.   For novice exercisers, the following questions and answers will help you use your heart rate as a guide to your exercise intensity:

• *How do I measure my heart rate during exercise?* The same way as at rest—by taking your pulse. (See Appendix A.)

• *How often during exercise should I calculate my heart rate?* Initially, you may need to check your heart rate as often as every 5 minutes. Once you are familiar with your own appropriate exercise intensity, though, you'll probably only need to do it a few times each workout. I generally recommend that you check your rate at the following times:

1. *Before starting to exercise.* If it is above 100 beats per minute and remains this high after 15 minutes or so of rest, don't exercise at all.
2. *After you complete your warm-up.* If your heart rate is above your heart rate limit at this point, slow down until it drops below the limit. In this situation you performed your warm-up at too high an intensity. Start off slower next time.
3. *After you've been exercising at your peak intensity for about 5 minutes.* If it is above your limit, slow down and recheck it within 5 minutes.
4. *At the point when you stop the aerobic phase and begin your cool-down.*
5. *When you complete your cool-down.* If your heart rate isn't below 100 beats per minute, rest until it reaches this level. Only then take a shower or drive off in your car.

• *Can I rely on a portable heart rate monitor instead of checking my heart rate manually?* Commercially available meters generally are worn on the chest and provide continual monitoring of your heart rate by transmitting electrical signals to a special wristwatch or a computer that's also worn on your chest. You can usually program your heart rate limit into the device and it will set off an alarm if you exceed it. Provided you purchase a reliable model, such monitors can be a valuable aid, although they're certainly not a necessity. Consult a member of your health-care team before purchasing one. Ask him or her which type is more accurate. Then before you actually purchase a specific one, ask that team member to help you verify its accuracy while you're wearing it.

Perceived Exertion. One of the simplest ways to quantify your exercise intensity is to use the scale I've reproduced in Table 3.1 (see p. 64). Named after its originator, the Swedish exercise physiologist Dr. Gunnar Borg who developed it in the early 1950s, the Borg scale helps you judge your exercise intensity based on your on-the-spot perception of how hard the exercise feels.[16] This "rating of perceived exertion" (or RPE) is outlined on a scale from 6 to 20, which you consult as you exercise. If you're exerting yourself at a level that you feel is fairly strenuous, you might assign your effort an RPE of 13. When you reach the all-out huffing-and-puffing stage, you would choose a much higher rating of about 17.

Generally, an RPE of 12 to 13 corresponds to an exercise intensity of 60% to 75% of the maximal heart rate. In other words, the 12-to-13 RPE range corresponds to your training target heart rate zone, which is what you want to aim for during the aerobic portion of your workout. Unless you're a competitive athlete and your doctor has given the okay, never exceed a score of 15—even if your heart rate is below your prescribed limit.

You should use ideally both your heart rate and RPE to monitor the intensity of your workouts. However, provided your doctor has assured you that you do not suffer from cardiovascular disease (such as coronary artery disease), you may rely entirely on your RPE, should you wish.

Basic Aerobic Exercises to Get You Started

No, aerobic exercises *don't* require excessive speed or strength, but they *do* require that you place demands on your cardiovascular system to supply your muscles with oxygen for energy production. In contrast, "*anaerobic*" exercise, as the prefix implies, means "without oxygen." Sprinting is an anaerobic activity. It involves an all-out burst of effort and relies on metabolic processes that do not require oxygen for energy production. Such processes result in fatigue within a relatively short time.

Aerobic exercise is far better than anaerobic for people with arthritis who want to improve their health, for these reasons: Energy expenditure is related to how much oxygen your working muscles use during exercise. Aerobic exercise obviously uses up more oxygen than anaerobic exercise. Also, because it's more moderate and you can do it longer, aerobic exercise allows you to expend far more energy than anaerobic exercise. Furthermore, when you exercise aerobically, you can better monitor your heart rate and keep it within your prescribed limit. Anaerobic exercise is more likely to push your heart rate above

Basic aerobic exercises

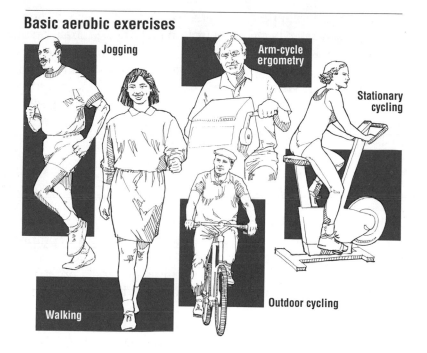

Jogging

Arm-cycle ergometry

Stationary cycling

Walking

Outdoor cycling

that limit, which can be dangerous if you have cardiovascular disease. Finally, anaerobic exercise is likely to place more stress on your musculoskeletal system than aerobic exercise.

The beginning aerobic exercises I recommend most for arthritis patients whose joint pain or inflammation is mild (or absent) are walking, cycling, and, for those in functional capacity classes 1 and 2, jogging. Each has its advantages and disadvantages:

Walking.   Most experts, including me, consider walking one of the most appropriate aerobic activities for many arthritis patients.[17] It's simple and straightforward, requiring no special skill, setting, or equipment except a good pair of shoes. Walking is one of the exercises least likely to cause or aggravate musculoskeletal problems. The intensity is easy to control; many people with systemic arthritis manifestations or other chronic diseases, such as coronary artery disease, can walk and get the desired conditioning effect. And the findings of a recent study, conducted by Drs. Tom R. Thomas and Ben R. Londeree, suggest that at fast speeds the energy expenditure for walking approaches that for jogging.[18]

If your arthritis affects one or more of your weight-bearing joints—your ankles, knees, hips, or spine—you'll probably have a tendency to compensate by adopting an unnatural walking gait. Such compensations should be avoided because they often place added strain on other joints. In their book *Walking Medicine*, Gary Yanker and Kathy Burton recommend that rather than limping, which involves taking a shorter step with the leg that's more affected by arthritis and a longer stride with the one that isn't, you might take shorter steps with both legs. As you become more and more accustomed to walking, you should then gradually increase your stride length with both legs.[19]

Jogging. The advantages of jogging are similar to those for walking. The catch is that during jogging, your feet strike the ground with a force that's usually equal to 3 to 4 times your body weight. This force is transmitted to your weight-bearing joints and, over time and done to excess, could worsen the arthritis in those locations. In contrast to jogging, walking exerts only a force of 1 to 1-1/2 times your weight on the weight-bearing joints.[19] Jogging requires generally greater exertion—or intensity—than walking, thus it often induces a heart rate that exceeds your designated limit. However, if you're enthusiastic about jogging, despite the greater risks that may accompany it, I recommend that it be preceded by a walking program, then by a walk-jog regimen. Many patients with milder degrees of arthritis are eventually able to include jogging in their training program with a great deal of success, when they approach their exercise regimen in a sensible manner.

Stationary Cycling. This is an activity busy people love. While you're pedaling away on your stationary cycle (also known as a "cycle ergometer"), you can do other things, such as read or watch TV. Stationary cycling gives you no excuse for not exercising should the weather make outdoor cycling impossible, and it causes less wear and tear on the musculoskeletal system than many aerobic activities, including walking. To reduce the stress on your knees, be sure to set the saddle height so that your knee joints almost fully straighten during pedaling.

There is a disadvantage, though. During a long ride, you may find you develop sore buttocks. This can be especially troublesome for people whose sacroiliac (or tailbone) joints are affected by arthritis, such as those with ankylosing spondylitis. For such reasons, I often have patients combine stationary cycling with walking.

Some stationary cycles, such as the Schwinn Air-Dyne, are a variation on the theme. They help you achieve higher energy expenditures by working your arms and legs simultaneously. You pump your legs up and down while you move your arms forward and back. The result is a more thorough upper- and lower-body workout with less stress on your lower-limb joints. I recommend these cycle ergometers for many of our arthritis patients, especially those who use their arms a lot in their occupations or for recreation. If you have arthritis in your hand or finger joints, be sure not to grip the handles of the bike too firmly. And if pulling with your arms causes discomfort, use them only for pushing (or vice versa).

Arm-Cycle Ergometry. This is one alternative for patients whose lower-limb arthritis problems prevent them from using their legs during exercise but whose arms are relatively unaffected. There is a downside to arm-cycle ergometry. Because the upper-limb muscles are smaller than those of the lower limb, you have to work far harder to achieve a given energy expenditure.

Outdoor Cycling. Outdoor cycling can be far more enjoyable and exhilarating than indoor cycling. The disadvantage over a stationary workout is that roads tend to go up and down. An unexpected incline could place excessive stress on your knee joints or cause an excessive elevation in your heart rate. Also, too many downhill stretches and excessive delays in traffic and at stoplights may lessen considerably your energy expenditure, thus forcing you to increase the duration of your workout in order to gain your desired energy expenditure. Then there is the danger that traffic poses. Still, if you can eliminate some of these drawbacks, outdoor cycling is great.

Aerobic Exercise Recommendations for People With Moderate to Severe Pain, Inflammation, or Poor Functional Capacity

For someone with arthritis, aerobic exercise is a touchier and more complex issue than range-of-motion and even muscle-strengthening exercise. I believe this segment of your workout is the most important for conferring major health benefits (in particular, preventing heart disease). And so this book is designed to give those of you with moderate to severe arthritis symptoms or a substantial limitation in your functional capacity the maximum amount of guidance about how to proceed safely.

What should you do when you've been exercising for awhile with only mild arthritis symptoms, and then suddenly your joint malady flares up? Or here's another scenario: You haven't started aerobic exercise yet and are wondering whether you can because you're in steady pain and bothered constantly by the tell-tale inflammatory signs of joint pain, warmth, redness, or swelling.

My recommendations about safe exercise—including a medical questionnaire designed to screen out those of you who shouldn't start the programs outlined in this book without the express permission of your doctor—are contained in chapter 5. I've found that many arthritis patients are so dependent on exercise to make them feel better that, even with moderate to severe pain and signs of inflammation, they'd rather use innovative ways to make exercise possible than to give it up entirely. Here are some of the things they do:

First, they consult Table 5.1 (page 107) called "Joints Stressed by Aerobic Activities" to find other forms of aerobics that will not involve the use of affected joints. For example, people with osteoarthritis of their knees or hips who do weight-bearing forms of exercise that cause pain would discover, by consulting this box, that swimming, aqua-aerobics, or arm-cycle ergometry may be the answer to their aggravated pain problems. The latter types of exercise are much less likely to trigger pain in the knees and hips.

Having said this, I must also emphasize that there are times when simply changing forms of exercise won't work. During a flare-up of rheumatoid arthritis in which many joints are throbbing and inflamed, it may be advisable to omit aerobics entirely from your exercise schedule for the time being. Until you get your symptoms under control, just do daily gentle range-of-motion and isometric strengthening exercises, which place minimal stress on joints.

A second approach is to rotate the types of aerobic exercise you do so that different parts of your body are being used and there is less stress on a few joints. This is known as "cross-training." For example, instead of just walking briskly for 40 minutes, you might try walking for 20 minutes and then stationary cycling for the remaining 20. Or should you develop knee pain while you're cycling on a Schwinn Air-Dyne, you might switch from leg propulsion to arm locomotion. Once the pain in your knees subsides, you could resume using your legs, but at a lower intensity. A 4-day-a-week walker with leg pain might alternate between walking one day and cycling the next.

In other words, experiment. Try different exercise configurations. Whatever works best for you is what you should do. Cross-training is an injury-prevention strategy that many competitive athletes find useful. It can easily be adopted by arthritis patients (and any regular exerciser in the peak of health) to prevent injury.

A third possibility is "interval training." This means doing a series of bouts of exercise, each separated by a short rest period. Interval training takes the place of one long, endurance-oriented workout.

Here's how this might work: Instead of cycling for 30 minutes without stopping, divide the session into 6 minisessions. Cycle for 5 minutes, then either cycle at a very low intensity or rest completely for 1 minute in between each minisession. The objective is to reduce temporarily the stress on your joints and relieve any undue fatigue you may be experiencing. Note that low-intensity cycling is preferable to a complete stop because abrupt cessation of exertion predisposes you to a dangerous drop in blood pressure.

Finally, you always have the option of reducing the overall intensity of your workout. No matter what exercise you're doing, this is almost guaranteed to lower joint stress. In one study, rheumatoid arthritis patients were told to exercise on their stationary cycles with little or no load during periods when their arthritis pain flared up.[20] This helped them maintain joint mobility and retain the habit of exercise without exacerbating their symptoms. Likewise, I encourage you to be creative about exercise. When pain and inflammation are more annoying than usual, find ways to transform higher intensity, more stressful aerobic activities into ones of lower stress.

The final approaches, interval training and a reduction in exercise intensity, are of great value to very sedentary persons and those in functional capacity class 3 (see box on page 15) who embark on aerobic exercise programs. I encourage you to use them.

PUTTING ON THOSE WALKING SHOES AND VENTURING FORTH

Here are guidelines for beginning a walking, walk-jog, or stationary cycling exercise program. The idea of each program is to ease your way gradually into the routine of regular exercise. After you've completed an introductory 8 weeks or so following one of the programs below, you'll be ready to start earning the 50 to 100 exercise health points discussed in the next chapter.

Please note that these programs are only intended as a guideline. Your individual circumstances may require you to progress more slowly than suggested.

Beginning Walking Program

Walking is a wonderful way for arthritis patients to get moving down the road to optimal health. But before you begin, you ideally should know your maximal MET value in order to estimate the speed (in mph

Making exercise possible when pain flares up

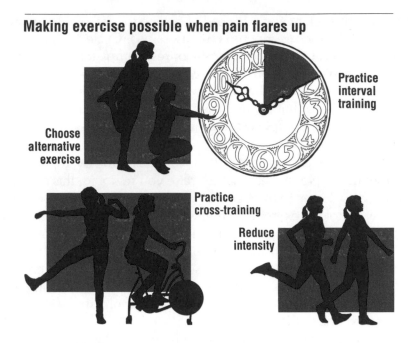

Choose alternative exercise

Practice interval training

Practice cross-training

Reduce intensity

or kph) at which you should walk during your first 8 weeks of exercise. Maximal MET value varies from one person to the next depending on his or her fitness level. If you've undergone an exercise test—which I urge our arthritis patients to do—your doctor should be able to provide you with your maximal MET value. If not, err on the side of caution and start out at a comfortable speed that does not exceed what's recommended in Table 3.2 on page 65 for a person with a maximal MET value of 6. Regardless of whether or not you know your maximal MET value, I strongly advise against exceeding 75% of your maximal heart rate and an RPE of 13 during these initial weeks. Table 3.2 shows what your estimated beginning walking speed should be. Using this table, Cheryl Lewis, whose maximal MET value was 5, started her walking program at a speed of about 2.6 mph or 4.2 kph.

The box on page 65 shows you what your walking program will look like in terms of each workout's duration and frequency.

Follow-Up Walk-Jog Program

Don't try jogging until you've followed a walking regimen for at least 6 weeks, ideally 12. You should be walking at a speed of at least 4 mph just before you graduate to jogging. If you're walking at a slower rate, you might as well stay with walking. Here are some pointers:

- When you start to jog, you should do so at a speed no faster than that at which you currently walk—and remember not to exceed the heart rate and RPE guidelines outlined earlier in this chapter.
- As always, warm up and cool down—each for at least 5 minutes. For the warm-up phase, walk briskly and try to raise gradually your heart rate to within at least 20 beats per minute of your target heart rate. Upon completing your jog, reduce gradually your speed to a slow walk over at least a 5-minute period.

The box on page 66 shows duration and frequency recommendations for your walk-jog program.

Beginning Stationary Cycling Program

If indoor cycling is more to your liking than walking, that's fine, for it's an excellent form of exercise.

Before you begin, you need to know your maximal MET value and your weight in either pounds or kilograms (choose the weight closest to yours in Table 3.3). If you haven't had an exercise test and don't know your maximal MET value, start out at a comfortable work rate that does not exceed that recommended for a person with a maximal MET value of 7. Regardless of whether or not you know your maximal MET value, I strongly advise against exceeding 75% of your maximal heart rate and an RPE of 13 during these initial weeks. Table 3.3 on page 68 shows your estimated beginning work rate for a stationary cycling program. Alan Hoffman, who weighed 220 pounds (100 kilograms) and had a maximal MET value of 7, began his cycling program at 93 watts.

The duration and frequency recommendations for the first 8 weeks of the cycling program are shown in the box on page 68.

Beginning Schwinn Air-Dyne Cycling Program

A second form of indoor cycling, which works both your arms and legs, is the Schwinn Air-Dyne, another good choice for your early attempts to form a regular exercise habit. Table 3.4 shows how to estimate your work load for the first 8 weeks. If you don't know your maximal MET value, use a value of no more than 7. Regardless of whether or not you know your maximal MET value, I strongly advise against exceeding 75% of your maximal heart rate and an RPE of 13 during these initial weeks. If you weigh 154 pounds (70 kilograms) and have a maximal MET value of 7, you would see by looking at Table 3.4 (page 69) that you should begin your Schwinn Air-Dyne cycling program at a work load of 1.3.

The box on page 69 shows duration and frequency recommendations for your Schwinn Air-Dyne program. Please be aware that there are a variety of other superb cycle ergometers that enable you to work your arms and legs simultaneously. Should you prefer to use one of them, these recommendations are equally applicable.

Beginning Program of Combined Walking and Stationary Cycling Using the Schwinn Air-Dyne

For people who get bored doing the same exercise day after day, I've devised an 8-week regimen that combines walking with cycling on the Schwinn Air-Dyne. This combination will also help reduce risk of injury.

The guidelines for walking and Schwinn Air-Dyne workouts apply to this program. Estimate your starting walking speed and Schwinn Air-Dyne work load for the first 8 weeks using Tables 3.2 and 3.4.

You may start with either activity. As always, warm up for 5 minutes. After completing the first activity, proceed immediately to the other one—no second warm-up is needed. When you finish, cool down for 5 minutes.

The duration and frequency recommendations for your combined walking and Schwinn Air-Dyne program are shown on page 70.

THAT ALL-IMPORTANT TRAINING LOG

I encourage our arthritis patients to use a training log to keep track of their exercise efforts, at least in the beginning. A log provides you and your doctor with helpful data. Moreover, it will help you be consistent with your exercise program. Following is an empty training log page. Make a number of photocopies of it and put them in a looseleaf notebook. Fill in a page after each day's worth of exercise. I also recommend that you include a copy of the Borg Perceived Exertion Scale (see Table 3.1, page 64) and the Arthritis Pain-Rating Scale (see page 109) in the front of your training log for easy reference.

DAILY EXERCISE TRAINING LOG

Date _____ Time of day _____ Body weight _____

Where I worked out _____

Resting pulse _____

Pre-exercise arthritis pain rating _____

Post-exercise arthritis pain rating _____

2-hour post-exercise arthritis pain rating _____

Pain accompanied by warmth, redness,
    or swelling?   Yes ___ No ___

Duration of range-of-motion, stretching, & muscle-
    strengthening portion of my workout _____

Pulse rate after range-of-motion, stretching, & muscle-
    strengthening portion of my workout
    (in beats per minute) _____

Aerobic workout

    Type of exercise _____

    Duration (in minutes) _____

    Distance covered or work rate/load _____

    Highest heart rate _____

    Borg RPE (at most intense part of workout) _____

    Any symptoms experienced _____

Enjoyment rating   ___ 1 Very unenjoyable

                    ___ 2 Unenjoyable

                    ___ 3 Somewhat unenjoyable

                    ___ 4 Enjoyable

                    ___ 5 Very enjoyable

Health points earned (see chapter 4) _____

Table 3.1
Borg Perceived Exertion Scale

The original Borg system for rating physical exertion is based on an open-ended scale running from 6 (equal to exertion at rest) to 20 (extreme effort).

Rating of perceived exertion or RPE	Verbal description of RPE
6	
7	Very, very light
8	
9	Very light
10	
11	Fairly light
12	
13	Somewhat hard
14	
15	Hard
16	
17	Very hard
18	
19	Very, very hard
20	

Note. From G.A. Borg, "Psychophysical Bases of Perceived Exertion," *Medicine and Science in Sports and Exercise*, *14*, pp. 377-387, 1982, © by The American College of Sports Medicine. Reprinted by permission.

Table 3.2
Estimated Speed at Which to Begin a Walking Program

Maximal MET value	Estimated walking speed (miles per hour)	Estimated walking speed (kilometers per hour)
4	1.8 mph	2.9 kph
5	2.6 mph	4.2 kph
6	3.4 mph	5.4 kph
7 and above	4 mph	6.4 kph

Walking Program		
Week	**Duration per session**	**Frequency per week**
1	10 minutes	3-5 times
2	15 minutes	3-5 times
3	20 minutes	3-5 times
4	25 minutes	3-5 times
5	30 minutes	3-5 times
6	35 minutes	3-5 times
7	40 minutes	3-5 times
8	45 minutes	3-5 times
9 and onward	It's time to start earning those 50 to 100 health points a week. Keep your exercise time at 45 minutes per session and gradually increase your speed until you exceed 60% of your maximal heart rate (if you are not doing so yet). If this does not result in the desired weekly energy expenditure using the health points charts in chapter 4,* do one or more of the following: Try exercising within the upper range of your target heart rate zone; exercise more frequently; or increase the duration of each exercise session.	

*At fast speeds, the energy you expend for walking approaches that for jogging. Therefore, for speeds of 4 mph (or 6.4 kph) or faster, I recommend that you use our jogging chart in chapter 4 to calculate your health points.

Walk-Jog Program		
Week	**Duration per session**	**Frequency per week**
1	*20 minutes total*—Walk 4.5 min, jog 0.5 min, walk 4.5 min, jog 0.5 min, walk 4.5 min, jog 0.5 min, walk 4.5 min, jog 0.5 min*	3-5 times
2	*20 minutes total*—Walk 4 min, jog 1 min, walk 4 min, jog 1 min, walk 4 min, jog 1 min, walk 4 min, jog 1 min*	3-5 times
3	*20 minutes total*—Walk 3 min, jog 2 min, walk 3 min, jog 2 min, walk 3 min, jog 2 min, walk 3 min, jog 2 min*	3-5 times
4	*20 minutes total*—Walk 2 min, jog 3 min, walk 2 min, jog 3 min, walk 2 min, jog 3 min, walk 2 min, jog 3 min*	3-5 times
5	*20 minutes total*—Walk 5 min, jog 5 min, walk 5 min, jog 5 min*	3-5 times
6	*20 minutes total*—Walk 4 min, jog 6 min, walk 4 min, jog 6 min*	3-5 times
7	*20 minutes total*—Walk 3 min, jog 7 min, walk 3 min, jog 7 min*	3-5 times

(Cont.)

Walk-Jog Program (Continued)		
Week	Duration per session	Frequency per week
8	*20 minutes total*—Jog 10 min, walk 10 min*	3-5 times
9	*20 minutes total*—Jog 12 min, walk 8 min*	3-5 times
10	*20 minutes total*—Jog 15 min, walk 5 min*	3-5 times
11	*20 minutes total*—Jog 17 min, walk 3 min*	3-5 times
12	*20 minutes total*—Jog 20 min*	3-5 times
13 and onward	By the time you reach this point, you are likely to have exceeded 60% of your maximal heart rate; and you've possibly attained your desired weekly energy expenditure—100 health points per week using the health points charts in chapter 4.* If so, just keep following week 12's regimen. If, on the other hand, you haven't been able to exceed 60% of your maximal heart rate, increase your speed. If that does not result in 100 weekly health points, do one or more of the following: Try exercising within the upper range of your target heart rate zone; exercise more frequently; or increase the duration of each exercise session.	

*You may find that you are below your desired weekly energy expenditure during the early weeks of this walk-jog effort. You can compensate by walking longer at the end of the jogging phase, before starting your cool-down. Use the jogging chart in chapter 4 when calculating your health points for your walk-jog program.

Table 3.3
**Estimated Work Rate at Which to Begin
a Stationary Cycling (Legs Only) Program**

	Work rate (watts)					
Maximal MET value	Body weight = 110 lb (50 kg)	Body weight = 132 lb (60 kg)	Body weight = 154 lb (70 kg)	Body weight = 176 lb (80 kg)	Body weight = 198 lb (90 kg)	Body weight = 220 lb (100 kg)
4	20	25	29	33	37	41
5	29	35	41	47	53	58
6	38	46	53	61	68	76
7	47	56	65	75	84	93
8 and above	55	67	78	89	100	111

Stationary Cycling Program		
Week	**Duration per session**	**Frequency per week**
1	7.5 minutes	3-5 times
2	10 minutes	3-5 times
3	12.5 minutes	3-5 times
4	15 minutes	3-5 times
5	17.5 minutes	3-5 times
6	20 minutes	3-5 times
7	25 minutes	3-5 times
8	30 minutes	3-5 times
9 and onward	It's time to start earning those 50 to 100 health points a week. Keep your exercise time at 30 minutes per session and gradually increase your work rate until you exceed 60% of your maximal heart rate (if you are not doing so yet). If this does not result in the desired weekly energy expenditure using the health points charts in chapter 4, do one or more of the following: Try exercising within the upper range of your target heart rate zone; exercise more frequently; or increase the duration of each exercise session.	

Table 3.4
**Estimated Work Load at Which to Begin
a Schwinn Air-Dyne Cycling Program**

	Work load					
Maximal MET value	Body weight = 110 lb (50 kg)	Body weight = 132 lb (60 kg)	Body weight = 154 lb (70 kg)	Body weight = 176 lb (80 kg)	Body weight = 198 lb (90 kg)	Body weight = 220 lb (100 kg)
4	.4	.5	.6	.7	.7	.8
5	.6	.7	.8	.9	1.1	1.2
6	.8	.9	1.1	1.2	1.4	1.5
7	.9	1.1	1.3	1.5	1.7	1.9
8 and above	1.1	1.3	1.6	1.8	2	2.2

Schwinn Air-Dyne Program		
Week	**Duration per session**	**Frequency per week**
1	7.5 minutes	3-5 times
2	10 minutes	3-5 times
3	12.5 minutes	3-5 times
4	15 minutes	3-5 times
5	17.5 minutes	3-5 times
6	20 minutes	3-5 times
7	25 minutes	3-5 times
8	30 minutes	3-5 times
9 and onward	It's time to start earning those 50 to 100 health points a week. Keep your exercise time at 30 minutes per session and gradually increase your work load until you exceed 60% of your maximal heart rate (if you are not doing so yet). If this does not result in the desired weekly energy expenditure using the health points charts in chapter 4, do one or more of the following: Try exercising within the upper range of your target heart rate zone; exercise more frequently; or increase the duration of each exercise session.	

Combined Walking and Schwinn Air-Dyne Program

| Week | Duration per session | | Frequency per week |
	Walking	Schwinn Air-Dyne	
1	5 minutes	5 minutes	3-5 times
2	7.5 minutes	7.5 minutes	3-5 times
3	10 minutes	10 minutes	3-5 times
4	12.5 minutes	12.5 minutes	3-5 times
5	15 minutes	15 minutes	3-5 times
6	17.5 minutes	17.5 minutes	3-5 times
7	20 minutes	20 minutes	3-5 times
8	22.5 minutes	22.5 minutes	3-5 times
9 and onward	It's time to start earning those 50 to 100 health points a week. Keep the combined exercise time at 45 minutes per session and gradually increase the intensity until you exceed 60% of your maximal heart rate (if you're not doing so yet). If this does not result in the desired weekly energy expenditure using the health points charts in chapter 4, do one or more of the following: Try exercising within the upper range of your target heart rate zone; exercise more frequently; or increase the duration of each exercise session.		

Chapter 3
Prescription

☐ Start your exercise program slowly and progress gradually, as your condition permits.

☐ Always include a warm-up and cool-down in your exercise sessions—each at least 5 minutes long.

☐ Do range-of-motion, stretching, and aerobic exercises 3 to 5 times each week.

☐ Include muscle-strengthening exercises in your exercise routines 2 to 3 times each week.

☐ Aim for an exercise intensity that raises your heart rate to between 60% and 75% of your maximal value and elicits an RPE of 12 to 13 during the aerobic portion of your workout.

☐ Don't exceed 85% of your maximal heart rate or an RPE of 15 at any point in your workout.

☐ Exercise your options—choose aerobic exercises that are convenient and appropriate for your arthritis.

☐ Make use of cross-training and interval training.

☐ When your arthritis flares up, de-intensify your workouts.

Chapter 4

The Health Points System: Insuring Maximum Health Benefits With Minimum Risk

In trying to motivate arthritis patients to follow exercise prescriptions, I always feel I'm walking several fine lines. First, as a physician, I have to educate patients adequately so their excuse can never be "I didn't understand." Then I must alert them to the seriousness of their condition and the risks involved in exercise without making them feel it's hopeless. And, most importantly, I have to impress on patients the fact that drugs and medical care can go only so far in making them well. They must do the rest by making positive lifestyle changes, including regular exercise. With our Health Points System, you can chart how effective your exercise program is likely to be in promoting your health.*

---

*Those of you with mild arthritis have the option of following Ken Cooper's well-known Aerobic Point System instead of our Health Points System. He describes it fully in *The Aerobics Program for Total Well-Being*.[1]

We devised the Health Points System so that our patients will do just enough exercise to gain optimal health benefits without exerting themselves to the point where exercise becomes risky. The system incorporates these two goals—effectiveness and safety. As a person with arthritis, you must strike a delicate balance between them.

As I explained in chapter 3, our system is based on the number of calories people of various weights expend during exercise. From my and other doctors' and exercise physiologists' experience and studies, it is now known that

aerobic exercise performed for 15 to 60 minutes per workout 3 to 5 days each week at an intensity that raises the heart rate to between 60% and 85% of the maximal value will result in an energy expenditure that brings about the desired health benefits.

HOW THE HEALTH POINTS SYSTEM WORKS

If you're a novice exerciser, you should consider following one of the beginning exercise programs I outlined in chapter 3 to work your body up to an appropriate level of exertion gradually over 8 weeks or so (and more if necessary). Although you can start using the Weekly Health Points Exercise Tally Sheet (see page 75) during this time, you should not try specifically to earn 50 to 100 health points until you reach week 9. Then start aiming for 50 to 100 health points each week. The precise number of points you should strive for depends on the degree of arthritis pain you are experiencing, the presence or absence of inflammatory signs, and your current functional capacity; recommendations that take these factors into consideration are summarized toward the end of chapter 5.

In many aspects of life, we like to know where we stand in our endeavors, to get "report cards." Our Health Points System is a kind of report card on your exercise program. But you fill it out, not a doctor or a teacher. The system lets you quantify one constructive lifestyle change—regular aerobic exercise—that you can easily undertake to improve your health and reduce your risk of developing serious chronic arthritis complications. By charting your progress, you can see clearly what you are accomplishing and where you stand.

Please note: Our Health Points System is intended for those with mild or no joint pain or inflammation who are in functional capacity classes 1 and 2—and if not too severely limited by your arthritis,

WEEKLY HEALTH POINTS EXERCISE TALLY SHEET

Your Weekly Goal: To earn between 50 and 100 health points each week, which corresponds to an expenditure of 10 to 20 calories per kilogram (2.2 pounds) of body weight per week. Exceeding this upper limit does not provide substantially more health benefit; thus you should keep your weekly health points total at, or very near, 100. To gain optimal benefit, you should earn your weekly quota of points across at least 3 workouts.

To find out how many health points you earned during an exercise session, simply use the chart (see Tables 4.1-4.5, pages 88-95) that corresponds to the form of aerobic exercise you're doing and fill in the results below:

Monday   Tuesday   Wednesday   Thursday   Friday   Saturday   Sunday   Total weekly health points

_____ pt. + _____ pt. + _____ pt. + _____ pt. + _____ pt. + _____ pt. + _____ pt. = _____ pt.

(100 pt. maximum)

INTERPRETING THE EFFECTIVENESS OF YOUR WEEKLY EXERCISE EFFORT*

100 health points from exercise	Ideal. *You couldn't do better!*
70-99 health points from exercise	Very good. *Be proud of yourself.*
50-69 health points from exercise	Good. *But you could do better.*
20-49 health points from exercise	Fair. *Try a bit harder.*
10-19 health points from exercise	Poor. *Come on, now.*
Less than 10 health points from exercise	Very poor. *Need we say more?*

*If your arthritis or other medical conditions are such that you cannot attain the desired weekly number of health points, ignore this interpretation. Be proud of whatever progress you are able to make.

class 3. It's not intended for anyone suffering a severe arthritis flare-up, whose arthritis is characterized by severe symptoms in many joints most of the time, or who has joint damage/deformity/instability or other arthritis complications that severely limit functional capacity (that is, some patients in functional capacity class 3 and all in class 4).

Some types of arthritis—such as rheumatoid—tend to fluctuate. If your arthritis is flaring up, be realistic and honest with yourself, and either sit out aerobics for awhile or use some of the ways I outlined in chapter 3 to drastically modify and *de*-intensify your aerobics routine. To follow our Health Points System during such times could well be detrimental, rather than beneficial, to your health.

If you find your condition is such that you cannot attain the desired weekly number of health points, don't become worried or discouraged. Provided you perform some type of aerobic exercise—even one for which I don't provide a health points chart—for a minimum of 15 minutes at least 3 days a week, you'll derive important health-related benefits, to be sure. Rather than attempt to fulfill expectations that may be unrealistic given your present clinical circumstances, be proud of whatever progress you can make. Also keep in mind when referring to my interpretation of the effectiveness of your weekly exercise effort on the tally sheet that *it is not applicable to persons whose arthritis (as opposed to factors such as a lack of interest or desire, or a case of laziness) prevents them from attaining the recommended weekly number of health points*. This fact is of particular importance to those of you in functional capacity class 3 whose condition simply may not allow you to achieve 50 or more weekly points.

HOW TO USE
OUR HEALTH POINTS CHARTS

The only way people can get a truly accurate fix on their energy expenditure during exercise is through laboratory testing. Technicians can use sophisticated equipment to measure the exact amount of oxygen the body takes up during a workout. The charts that follow are derived from numerous exercise research studies performed in such laboratories.

The health points charts in this chapter (Tables 4.1-4.4) cover walking, jogging, stationary cycling, and the Schwinn Air-Dyne—all forms of exercise described in depth in chapter 3. It was possible to formulate charts for these forms of exercise because (a) none require much skill, and (b) there's a great deal of outstanding research data available for them.

If you're exercising on equipment that I have not provided charts for but which gives you a readout of the number of calories you've expended, you can also easily convert such a number to health points. Divide the read-out number (calories) by the number you get when you divide your body weight (in pounds) by 11. If your body weight is in kilograms, divide the read-out number by the number you get when you divide your kilogram weight by 5. For example, if the read-out number is 120 calories and you weigh 165 pounds (75 kilograms), you have earned 8 health points (165 pounds ÷ 11, or 75 kilograms ÷ 5, = 15 and 120 calories ÷ 15 = 8 health points).

To determine the health points you earn for walking and jogging, you need to know the distance you covered during your workout, and the time it took you. If you're lucky enough to have access to a measured running track, figuring the distance will pose no problem. Otherwise you might want to invest in a pedometer or use your car's odometer to stake out a stretch of road to use as a track. You'll need a watch with a second hand or a stopwatch to measure accurately the duration of your exercise session.

To ascertain your health points on the charts for stationary cycling and the Schwinn Air-Dyne, you'll need to know the duration of your workout, your work rate (wattage) or work load (for the Schwinn Air-Dyne), and your weight.

To show you how easy the Health Points System is to use, on pages 78 and 79 are some examples from Alan Hoffman's and Cheryl Lewis's training logs. Use the Tables 4.1-4.5 (found at the end of this chapter) to verify the number of health points they earned for each activity. At the time of these workouts, Alan's weight had decreased to 209 pounds (95 kilograms) while Cheryl's had increased to 136 pounds (62 kilograms).

OTHER AEROBIC EXERCISE CHOICES: THE PROS AND CONS

Table 4.5 (see p. 94) is a chart labeled "Other Aerobic Activities." In order to vary your routine, you may want to try some of these other forms of exercise. When doing so, keep in mind that these other forms of aerobic exercise either require skill, are influenced by external factors such as the weather or terrain, or have not been intensively

Alan

Date	Activity	Time	Distance/ work load	Health points	Notes
S					
M	Walk	22-1/2 min	1-1/2 miles	16	Walking felt good.
	Schwinn Air-Dyne	22-1/2 min	2.3 WL	11.3	
T					
W	Schwinn Air-Dyne	20 min	2.5 WL	11.6	Hips hurt before swimming, but felt okay later.
	Swimming	15 min	12 RPE	6.6	
T	Walk	25 min	1.7 miles	18.2	Walked farther today. A little sore, but okay.
	Schwinn Air-Dyne	20 min	2.5 WL	11.6	
F					
S	Walk	25 min	1.7 miles	18.2	Good workout.
	Swim	20 min	12 RPE	8.8	
				102.3	**Total: Week** 28

researched. Thus, although this table is extremely useful, it isn't as precise as those for walking, jogging, and stationary cycling. To use this table you need to know how long you exercised and whether you exercised at a light (RPE < 12), moderate (RPE = 12-13), or heavy (RPE > 13) intensity.

The ideal aerobic exercise for you has four basic characteristics:

Cheryl

Date	Activity	Time	Distance/ work load	Health points	Notes
S					
M	Walk	20 min	1 mile	6.5	No problems.
	Cycle (legs)	10 min	50 watts	5.0	
T	Cycle (legs)	15 min	50 watts	7.5	Tired after water aerobics.
	Aqua- aerobics	20 min	11 RPE	7.0	
W					
T	Cycle (legs)	15 min	50 watts	7.5	A little stiff before cycling.
	Aqua- aerobics	20 min	11 RPE	7.0	Felt good after water aerobics.
F	Walk	15 min	3/4 mile	4.5	Took it easy today because of
	Cycle (legs)	12-1/2 min	50 watts	6.3	flare-up, but still earned points!
S					
				51.3	**Total: Week** 28

- It's pleasant. An exercise you enjoy is one you're more likely to stick with.
- It is practical and fits into your lifestyle—something you can perform conveniently all year round.
- It uses large muscle groups. Why is this important? Because the larger the muscle groups involved in your exercise effort, the

greater your body's oxygen uptake and, hence, energy expenditure.

- It imposes the least possible stress on joints affected by arthritis. (In chapter 5, see Table 5.1, "Joints Stressed by Aerobic Activities.")

Here are the pros and cons of some specific aerobic exercise choices, other than those already discussed (in addition to these, there are many other aerobic exercises I don't cover here):

Swimming

This is an excellent aerobic activity because it incorporates both the upper and lower body musculature. And, because it's a nonweight-bearing activity, the chances of exacerbating your arthritis are extremely low—probably even lower than with cycling. Moreover, the warmth of the water may help relax you and reduce your arthritis pain. Indeed, swimming, and other forms of water exercise, are among the best aerobic choices for people with arthritis. Unfortunately, for many people swimming is not an option. It requires a pool and the means to get there. This is the only reason I didn't include it in the beginning aerobic exercise choices in chapter 3.

If you do opt for swimming, you may find it necessary occasionally to modify your swimming style in accordance with your arthritis. For example, in one study researchers found that people with arthritis of the neck vertebrae could not swim because their limited neck movement impeded effective breathing. However, after they were provided with snorkels and masks, many of these same people were able to participate in a regular swimming program.[2] Such creative solutions are likely to become more common as greater numbers of arthritis patients take up aerobic exercise programs.

The normal recommended pool temperature is 86 °F (or 30 °C). Temperatures should not exceed 100 °F (about 38 °C) because this reduces your capacity to perform aerobic exercise and may trigger cardiovascular problems.[3]

Aqua-Aerobics

This is just what the name implies—aerobic exercises done in water. When you do range-of-motion exercises under water, the water provides resistance and your strength may improve. Walking while partially submerged in water is another possibility; compared with walking on land, it places less stress on your weight-bearing joints.

As a general rule, water supports the percentage of the body submerged in it. In other words, a 132-pound (60-kilogram) person who is standing on a scale at the bottom of the pool and who is submerged in water up to his or her navel would get a reading of about 66 pounds (30 kilograms) on the scale. (Water to the navel means about 1/2 of the body is submerged, so 132 pounds × 1/2 = 66).[4] By varying the depth of the water that weight-bearing activities, such as walking, are performed in, it's possible to control the amount of stress placed on the joints. *Because water neutralizes gravity while providing resistance, this increasingly popular form of exercise allows you to increase your strength, flexibility, and aerobic fitness with a very low risk of worsening your arthritis.* Those of you who find the prospect of exercising in a swimming pool appealing can consult Ken Cooper's book, *Overcoming Hypertension*, for detailed guidelines.[5] If you live in the United States, I also recommend that you contact the Arthritis Foundation and ask about their aquatic programs.

Cross-Country Skiing

Ken Cooper rates this as the top aerobic activity. Ken's reasoning: "You have more muscles involved than just the legs; and any time you get more muscles involved, you get more aerobic benefit."[6] The heavy clothing you wear and the weighty equipment you must carry further enhance the aerobic effect (that is, your energy expenditure) over that of walking or jogging at similar speeds. Furthermore, it not only enables you to burn off calories in a highly efficient manner, but it's also a low-impact exercise that's unlikely to aggravate your arthritis.

There are drawbacks. The total exertion is greatly affected by variations in skill, snow surface, terrain, temperature and weather conditions, and altitude. Also, it's difficult to take your pulse in the middle of this activity. One way around these barriers is mechanical cross-country skiing devices, which some of our patients enjoy using. If you have arthritis of your hand or finger joints, do not grip the ski handles too tightly. Some people with severe arthritis of their upper limbs may find this exercise too difficult.

Stair Climbing

A testament to the current popularity of stair-climbing machines is that they always seem to be in use at health clubs. These machines let you simulate the act of climbing flights of stairs, thus allowing you to work the large muscles in your back, buttocks, and legs and expend large amounts of energy in a relatively short period of time.

People with arthritis of their knee joints should look elsewhere for an aerobic workout, for the stress stair climbing places on the knee joint is thought to be equivalent to lifting 4 to 6 times your body weight. Needless to say, it's likely to aggravate any existing problem in that area.[7] For similar reasons, people with arthritis of their hip or ankle joints may need to avoid stair climbing.

Rope Skipping

Most people with arthritis should probably avoid this high-impact activity, especially if they have arthritis of their weight-bearing joints. Those with arthritis of their fingers, hands, arms, and shoulders often find rope skipping difficult—if not impossible—to perform. Also, it's relatively strenuous and may result in excessively high heart rates. Even at that, for a given heart rate, the energy expenditure is not as high as that for some other strenuous aerobic exercises such as jogging.

Rebounding

This refers to running in place on a minitrampoline. The advantage of rebounding is the reduced risk for exacerbating your arthritis. However, your energy expenditure probably won't be great.[8] The trampoline serves as too much of a helpmate, causing your legs to spring up almost without any exertion on your part. This may be a suitable activity during the very early phase of your exercise program or when your arthritis pain is more than mild or accompanied by other evidence of inflammation, but it may have to be abandoned in favor of something more vigorous later on.

Aerobic Dance

Aerobic dancing is steady, rhythmic movements done to the beat of relatively fast music, usually rock. Benches that range in height from 6 to 12 inches (15 to 30 centimeters) have been introduced recently into aerobic dance workouts in an attempt to increase the exercise intensity while reducing the impact and risk of injury.[9] Unfortunately, traditional high-impact aerobics classes and even bench aerobics are not something I can recommend for most people with arthritis of their weight-bearing joints. Unless the class is specially designed for people with arthritis, even many low-impact aerobics classes are likely to place too much stress on arthritic joints. One viable alternative is to participate in the Arthritis Foundation's program "People With Arthritis Can Exercise," or PACE. These programs are now available in many cities in the United States and are also available in a videotaped version featuring professional golfer Jan Stephenson. I'm an enthusiastic supporter of these programs.

Circuit Resistance Training

This is a combination of aerobics and strength training. Typically, an exerciser would use a series of resistance training machines and move from one to another with very short rest periods in between (usually 15 to 30 seconds). Performed correctly, circuit training improves the cardiovascular system, builds and tones muscles, and burns calories during one carefully constructed workout.

Sounds great, doesn't it?

I didn't want to dismiss this exercise option out of hand so I reviewed the medical literature and did our own study of its possible rehabilitation benefits.[10] The catch is this: The primary benefit is enhancement of muscular strength, not improvement in the cardiovascular system. Thus, I do not recommend it for persons with arthritis unless it's performed in conjunction with other forms of aerobic exercise. Even then, you must be sure to adhere to the strength-training guidelines outlined in chapter 3.

Recreational Sports

People with relatively good control of joint inflammation—especially those in functional capacity classes 1 and 2—are capable of participating in many recreational sports. However, you may need to avoid sports that involve a lot of stopping and starting (e.g., tennis), sudden twisting and turning (e.g., racquetball), body contact (e.g., football), or high-impact activities (e.g., jumping). This is particularly true for people who have had joint replacements or have unstable joints. If you're determined to engage in recreational sports, you may have to modify the rules in order to minimize the impact on your joints. When performed in such a way, recreational sports can be—and often are—a very valuable component of an arthritis rehabilitation exercise program.

Although I have not included sample introductory programs for each of these alternative exercise choices, you should be able to use the walking and stationary cycling programs at the end of chapter 3 as prototypes for your own programs. For example, an introductory swimming program might be as follows:

Week	Duration per session	Frequency per week
1	7.5 minutes	3-5 times
2	10 minutes	3-5 times
3	12.5 minutes	3-5 times
4	15 minutes	3-5 times
5	17.5 minutes	3-5 times
6	20 minutes	3-5 times
7	25 minutes	3-5 times
8	30 minutes	3-5 times
9 and onward	It's time to start earning those 50 to 100 health points a week. Keep your exercise time at 30 minutes per session and gradually increase your swimming speed until you exceed 60% of your maximal heart rate (if you are not doing so yet). If this does not result in the desired weekly energy expenditure using the Other Aerobic Activities chart (Table 4.5, p. 94), do one or more of the following: Try exercising within the upper range of your target heart rate zone; exercise more frequently; or increase the duration of each exercise session.	

In using this swimming program, as with any aerobic exercise, begin at a comfortable intensity. During the initial weeks you would not exceed 75% of your maximal heart rate and an RPE of 13. You would also be sure to warm up and cool down—each for at least 5 minutes. This could be done with the use of slower swimming or other activities in the water.

Other aerobic choices

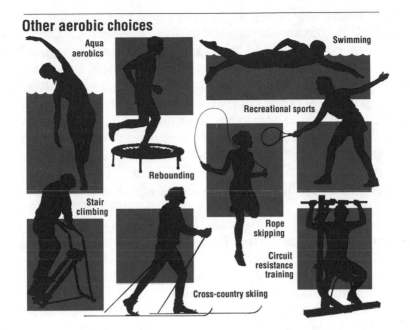

Aqua aerobics

Swimming

Recreational sports

Rebounding

Stair climbing

Rope skipping

Circuit resistance training

Cross-country skiing

THE FOUR-LETTER WORD
YOU MUST NOT UTTER

That word is "quit."

You've probably noticed that I keep pushing the notion of *regular* exercise—not sporadic exercise, not fair-weather exercise, but the kind of persistent exercise you engage in almost daily because it's a habit, like brushing your teeth. There's a reason. When you exercise, your body and its various organ systems are being exposed to potent physiologic stimuli. If you exercise on a regular basis at an appropriate intensity and duration, these stimuli result in specific adaptations your body makes that both enhance your ability to exercise and, at the same time, improve your health status. In other words, you'll be the happy recipient of all the benefits of a physically active lifestyle, benefits outlined in chapter 2.

Unfortunately, these benefits can't be stored up for a rainy day. They're reversible. All it takes to set this backtracking in motion is abstinence. If you stop training or reduce your level of physical activity below your required level, your body's systems soon readjust themselves to this diminished amount of physiologic stimuli. The end result: Those hard-won, exercise-related gains, which you worked so long and hard to achieve, are lost.

This "reversibility concept" is shown best in a landmark study of some 16,936 Harvard University alumni by Dr. Ralph S. Paffenbarger, Jr., and his colleagues.[11] In this study, many former college athletes became inactive adults. As a consequence, they were in worse shape—and at greater risk for cardiovascular disease—than their contemporaries who had not participated in sports in college but who had started exercising later in life. Researchers do not know how long it takes after you stop training before all the health benefits of exercise are lost. We do know that even after many years of training, a rapid decline in fitness occurs during the first 12 to 21 days of inactivity, and the fitness benefits of regular exercise are almost totally lost after 2 or 3 months.[12]

In view of this, it's imperative that you stick with your exercise program once you get started. This is easier said than done. A number of studies focusing on exercise compliance show that half or more of all patients drop out of their exercise program within a year and that the critical drop-out period is the first 3 to 6 months. You need motivators to get you through this critical time. The following suggestions will keep you huffing and puffing even when you'd rather be home in bed or watching television:

• *Make sure you fully understand the costs of not exercising versus the benefits of exercising.*

• *Start exercising slowly and progress gradually.* If you follow the beginning programs outlined in this book, this is just what you'll be doing.

• *Choose a form of exercise that's convenient as well as enjoyable.* Should you constantly score below a "4" on the enjoyment rating in the exercise log on page 63, your exercise program needs to be modified in some way.

• *Find a role model*—a friend, relative, or acquaintance who leads a physically active life. Find out why they love exercise so much.

• *Learn from your past exercise experiences.* Try to determine where you went wrong previously.

• *Obtain as much support for your exercise program as possible.* Enlist the company, or at the very least the moral support, of those closest to you. Keep in mind that health promotion should be a family affair. After all, your relatives are also at risk for developing arthritis and such maladies as heart disease. Point this out to your family and use it as the rationale to get as many of them as possible involved in your exercise program.

On the other hand, you must never let peer pressure force you to exercise more strenuously than you should. Always work at your own pace. You've got a special condition—arthritis—and even if your exercise companion has it too, his or her case won't necessarily be the same as yours. Though goals are important as exercise motivators, I urge you to keep yours realistic and modify them continually as your condition changes.

• *Bring your body to your place of exercise, even if your mind is temporarily on strike.* Often it's just a matter of overcoming mental inertia. A body at rest prefers to remain at rest. But once you start exercising, you may find you enjoy it more than you anticipated. Remember, special occasions, such as holidays or vacations, are no excuse.

• *Finally, remember that exercise lasts a lifetime.* A diamond may be forever, so they say in the beautiful, full-color advertisements for engagement rings. The same can be said about exercise, for physical activity is a lifelong pursuit.

I exhort you to do everything in your power to keep from becoming an exercise dropout, especially during the crucial initial months. Once you've passed the 6-month mark and tasted some of the tantalizing benefits of an active lifestyle, there's less and less chance you'll revert back to your unhealthy inactivity.

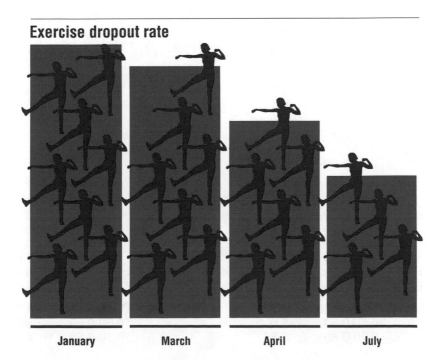

Exercise dropout rate

| January | March | April | July |

Table 4.1
Walking Health Points Chart

Time (min:sec)	Distance (miles)	Health points	Time (min:sec)	Distance (miles)	Health points
5:00	Under 0.10	0.8	7:30	Under 0.15	1.3
	0.10-0.14	1.0		0.15-0.19	1.5
	0.15-0.19	1.2		0.20-0.24	1.7
	0.20-0.24	1.4		0.25-0.29	1.9
	0.25-0.29	1.6		0.30-0.34	2.1
	0.30-0.33	1.8		0.35-0.39	2.3
	Over 0.33	*		0.40-0.44	2.5
				0.45-0.49	2.7
				Over 0.49	*
10:00	Under 0.20	1.7	12:30	Under 0.20	1.9
	0.20-0.24	1.8		0.20-0.29	2.3
	0.25-0.29	2.0		0.30-0.39	2.7
	0.30-0.34	2.2		0.40-0.49	3.1
	0.35-0.39	2.4		0.50-0.59	3.5
	0.40-0.44	2.6		0.60-0.69	3.9
	0.45-0.49	2.8		0.70-0.79	4.3
	0.50-0.54	3.0		0.80-0.83	4.7
	0.55-0.59	3.2		Over 0.83	*
	0.60-0.66	3.6			
	Over 0.66	*			
15:00	Under 0.30	2.5	17:30	Under 0.30	2.8
	0.30-0.39	2.9		0.30-0.49	3.5
	0.40-0.49	3.3		0.50-0.69	4.3
	0.50-0.59	3.7		0.70-0.89	5.1
	0.60-0.69	4.1		0.90-1.09	5.9
	0.70-0.79	4.5		1.10-1.16	6.7
	0.80-0.89	4.9		Over 1.16	*
	0.90-0.99	5.3			
	Over 0.99	*			
20:00	Under 0.40	3.4	22:30	Under 0.40	3.6
	0.40-0.59	4.1		0.40-0.59	4.4
	0.60-0.79	4.9		0.60-0.79	5.2
	0.80-0.99	5.7		0.80-0.99	6.0
	1.00-1.19	6.5		1.00-1.19	6.8
	1.20-1.33	7.3		1.20-1.39	7.6
	Over 1.33	*		1.40-1.49	8.4
				Over 1.49	*
25:00	Under 0.50	4.2	27:30	Under 0.50	4.5
	0.50-0.69	5.0		0.50-0.69	5.2
	0.70-0.89	5.8		0.70-0.89	6.0

Time (min:sec)	Distance (miles)	Health points	Time (min:sec)	Distance (miles)	Health points
25:00 (Cont.)			27:30 (Cont.)		
	0.90-1.09	6.6		0.90-1.09	6.8
	1.10-1.29	7.4		1.10-1.29	7.6
	1.30-1.49	8.2		1.30-1.49	8.4
	1.50-1.66	9.0		1.50-1.69	9.2
	Over 1.66	*		1.70-1.83	10.0
				Over 1.83	*
30:00	Under 0.50	4.6	35:00	Under 0.75	6.1
	0.50-0.74	5.6		0.75-0.99	7.0
	0.75-0.99	6.6		1.00-1.24	8.0
	1.00-1.24	7.6		1.25-1.49	9.0
	1.25-1.49	8.6		1.50-1.74	10.0
	1.50-1.74	9.6		1.75-1.99	11.0
	1.75-1.99	10.6		2.00-2.24	12.0
	Over 1.99	*		2.25-2.33	13.0
				Over 2.33	*
40:00	Under 1.00	7.5	45:00	Under 1.00	7.9
	1.00-1.24	8.5		1.00-1.49	9.9
	1.25-1.49	9.5		1.50-1.99	11.9
	1.50-1.74	10.5		2.00-2.49	13.9
	1.75-1.99	11.5		2.50-2.99	15.9
	2.00-2.24	12.5		Over 2.99	*
	2.25-2.49	13.5			
	2.50-2.66	14.5			
	Over 2.66	*			
50:00	Under 1.00	8.4	55:00	Under 1.00	8.8
	1.00-1.49	10.3		1.00-1.49	10.8
	1.50-1.99	12.4		1.50-1.99	12.8
	2.00-2.49	14.4		2.00-2.49	14.8
	2.50-2.99	16.4		2.50-2.99	16.8
	3.00-3.33	18.4		3.00-3.49	18.8
	Over 3.33	*		3.50-3.66	20.8
				Over 3.66	*
60:00	Under 1.00	9.3			
	1.00-1.49	11.2			
	1.50-1.99	13.2			
	2.00-2.49	15.2			
	2.50-2.99	17.2			
	3.00-3.49	19.2			
	3.50-3.99	21.2			
	Over 3.99	*			

*Use the Jogging Health Points Chart (Table 4.2).

Table 4.2
Jogging Health Points Chart

Time (min:sec)	Distance (miles)	Health points	Time (min:sec)	Distance (miles)	Health points
5:00	Under 0.40	3.6	7:30	Under 0.50	4.7
	0.40-0.49	4.4		0.50-0.59	5.4
	0.50-0.59	5.2		0.60-0.69	6.2
	0.60-0.69	6.0		0.70-0.79	7.0
	Over 0.69	6.8		0.80-0.89	7.8
				0.90-0.99	8.6
				1.00-1.09	9.4
				Over 1.09	10.2
10:00	Under 0.80	7.3	12:30	Under 1.00	9.2
	0.80-0.89	8.0		1.00-1.19	10.7
	0.90-0.99	8.8		1.20-1.39	12.3
	1.00-1.09	9.6		1.40-1.59	13.9
	1.10-1.19	10.4		1.60-1.79	15.5
	1.20-1.29	11.2		Over 1.79	17.1
	1.30-1.39	12.0			
	1.40-1.49	12.8			
	Over 1.49	13.6			
15:00	Under 1.20	10.9	17:30	Under 1.40	12.8
	1.20-1.39	12.5		1.40-1.59	14.3
	1.40-1.59	14.1		1.60-1.79	15.9
	1.60-1.79	15.7		1.80-1.99	17.5
	1.80-1.99	17.3		2.00-2.19	19.1
	2.00-2.19	18.9		2.20-2.39	20.7
	Over 2.19	20.5		2.40-2.59	22.4
				Over 2.59	24.0
20:00	Under 1.50	13.8	22:30	Under 1.75	16.0
	1.50-1.74	15.7		1.75-1.99	18.0
	1.75-1.99	17.7		2.00-2.24	20.0
	2.00-2.24	19.7		2.25-2.49	22.0
	2.25-2.49	21.7		2.50-2.74	24.0
	2.50-2.74	23.7		2.75-2.99	26.0
	2.75-2.99	25.7		3.00-3.24	28.0
	Over 2.99	27.7		Over 3.24	30.0
25:00	Under 2.00	18.2	27:30	Under 2.00	18.5
	2.00-2.24	20.2		2.00-2.24	20.4
	2.25-2.49	22.2		2.25-2.49	22.4
	2.50-2.74	24.2		2.50-2.74	24.4
	2.75-2.99	26.2		2.75-2.99	26.4
	3.00-3.24	28.2		3.00-3.24	28.4
	3.25-3.49	30.2		3.25-3.49	30.4

Time (min:sec)	Distance (miles)	Health points		Time (min:sec)	Distance (miles)	Health points
25:00 (Cont.)				27:30 (Cont.)		
	3.50-3.74	32.2			3.50-3.74	32.5
	Over 3.74	34.2			3.75-3.99	34.5
					Over 3.99	36.5
30:00	Under 2.50	22.7		35:00	Under 2.75	25.1
	2.50-2.74	24.6			2.75-2.99	27.0
	2.75-2.99	26.6			3.00-3.24	29.1
	3.00-3.24	28.6			3.25-3.49	31.1
	3.25-3.49	30.6			3.50-3.74	33.1
	3.50-3.74	32.6			3.75-3.99	35.1
	3.75-3.99	34.6			4.00-4.24	37.1
	4.00-4.24	36.6			4.25-4.49	39.1
	Over 4.24	38.6			4.50-4.74	41.1
					4.75-4.99	43.1
					Over 4.99	45.1
40:00	Under 3.00	27.6		45:00	Under 3.50	32.0
	3.00-3.49	31.5			3.50-3.99	35.9
	3.50-3.99	35.5			4.00-4.49	40.0
	4.00-4.49	39.5			4.50-4.99	44.0
	4.50-4.99	43.5			5.00-5.49	48.0
	5.00-5.49	47.5			5.50-5.99	52.0
	5.50-5.99	51.6			6.00-6.49	56.0
	Over 5.99	55.6			Over 6.49	60.0
50:00	Under 4.00	36.5		55:00	Under 4.50	40.9
	4.00-4.49	40.4			4.50-4.99	44.8
	4.50-4.99	44.4			5.00-5.49	48.9
	5.00-5.49	48.4			5.50-5.99	52.9
	5.50-5.99	52.4			6.00-6.49	56.9
	6.00-6.49	56.4			6.50-6.99	60.9
	6.50-6.99	60.4			7.00-7.49	64.9
	7.00-7.49	64.5			7.50-7.99	68.9
	Over 7.49	68.5			Over 7.99	72.9
60:00	Under 4.50	41.3				
	4.50-4.99	45.3				
	5.00-5.49	49.3				
	5.50-5.99	53.3				
	6.00-6.49	57.3				
	6.50-6.99	61.3				
	7.00-7.49	65.3				
	7.50-7.99	69.3				
	8.00-8.49	73.4				
	8.50-8.99	77.4				
	Over 8.99	81.4				

Table 4.3
Stationary Cycling (Legs Only) Health Points Chart

Work rate (watts)	Health points per minute							
	Under 100 lb	100 to 124 lb	125 to 149 lb	150 to 174 lb	175 to 199 lb	200 to 224 lb	225 to 249 lb	Over 249 lb
Under 25	0.34	0.28	0.24	0.22	0.20	0.18	0.17	0.16
25-49	0.54	0.44	0.36	0.32	0.28	0.26	0.24	0.22
50-74	0.76	0.60	0.50	0.42	0.38	0.34	0.32	0.30
75-99	0.98	0.76	0.62	0.54	0.48	0.42	0.38	0.36
100-124	1.20	0.92	0.76	0.64	0.56	0.50	0.46	0.42
125-149	1.42	1.10	0.90	0.76	0.66	0.58	0.54	0.48
150-174	1.64	1.26	1.02	0.86	0.76	0.68	0.60	0.56
175-199	1.86	1.42	1.16	0.98	0.84	0.76	0.68	0.62
200-224	2.08	1.58	1.28	1.08	0.94	0.84	0.76	0.68
225-249	2.30	1.76	1.42	1.20	1.04	0.92	0.82	0.76
Over 249	2.52	1.92	1.56	1.30	1.14	1.00	0.90	0.82

Table 4.4
Schwinn Air-Dyne Health Points Chart

Work load	Health points per minute							
	Under 100 lb	100 to 124 lb	125 to 149 lb	150 to 174 lb	175 to 199 lb	200 to 224 lb	225 to 249 lb	Over 249 lb
Under 0.5	0.34	0.28	0.24	0.22	0.20	0.18	0.17	0.16
0.5-0.9	0.52	0.40	0.34	0.30	0.26	0.24	0.22	0.21
1.0-1.4	0.74	0.56	0.48	0.40	0.36	0.32	0.30	0.28
1.5-1.9	0.96	0.74	0.60	0.52	0.46	0.42	0.38	0.34
2.0-2.4	1.18	0.90	0.74	0.62	0.56	0.50	0.44	0.42
2.5-2.9	1.40	1.06	0.86	0.74	0.64	0.58	0.52	0.48
3.0-3.4	1.62	1.22	1.00	0.84	0.74	0.66	0.60	0.54
3.5-3.9	1.84	1.40	1.14	0.96	0.84	0.74	0.66	0.62
4.0-4.4	2.06	1.56	1.26	1.06	0.92	0.82	0.74	0.68
4.5-4.9	2.28	1.72	1.40	1.18	1.02	0.90	0.82	0.74
Over 4.9	2.50	1.88	1.52	1.28	1.12	0.98	0.88	0.80

Table 4.5
Other Aerobic Activities

| Activity | Health points per minute | | |
| | Intensity* | | |
	Light	Moderate	Heavy
Aerobic dancing	0.35	0.53	0.79
Alpine skiing	0.35	0.53	0.70
Aqua-aerobics	0.35	0.53	0.79
Arm-cycle ergometry	0.22	0.35	0.61
Backpacking	0.53	0.70	0.88
(5% slope, 44 lb or 20 kg)			
4.0 mph (6.4 kph)	0.70		
4.5 mph (7.2 kph)	0.84		
5.0 mph (8.0 kph)	1.02		
6.0 mph (9.6 kph)	1.15		
7.0 mph (11.2 kph)	1.36		
Badminton	0.26	0.53	0.79
Ballet	0.44	0.53	0.70
Ballroom dancing	0.26	0.35	0.44
Baseball	0.26	0.35	0.44
Basketball	0.53	0.70	0.96
Bicycling	0.26	0.61	0.88
6.3 mph (10 kph)	0.42		
9.4 mph (15 kph)	0.52		
12.5 mph (20 kph)	0.62		
15.6 mph (25 kph)	0.74		
18.8 mph (30 kph)	0.86		
Canoeing	0.26	0.35	0.53
Catch (ball)	0.26	0.35	0.44
Circuit resistance training	0.26	0.44	0.61
Cricket	0.26	0.35	0.44
Cross-country skiing	0.44	0.79	1.14
2.5 mph (4 kph)	0.48		
3.8 mph (6 kph)	0.67		
5.0 mph (8 kph)	0.87		
6.3 mph (10 kph)	1.07		
7.5 mph (12 kph)	1.25		
8.8 mph (14 kph)	1.44		
Exercise classes	0.35	0.53	0.79
Fencing	0.44	0.61	0.88
Field hockey	0.53	0.70	0.88
Figure skating	0.35	0.53	0.88
Football (American)	0.44	0.53	0.61
Football (touch)	0.44	0.53	0.70

(Cont.)

Table 4.5
(Continued)

Activity	Health points per minute		
	Intensity*		
	Light	Moderate	Heavy
Golf			
Carrying clubs	0.45		
Pulling cart	0.35		
Riding cart	0.22		
Gymnastics		0.44	0.61	0.88
Handball (4-wall)		0.53	0.70	0.96
Hiking		0.26	0.53	0.70
Home calisthenics		0.26	0.44	0.70
Hunting		0.26	0.44	0.61
Ice hockey		0.53	0.70	0.88
Judo		0.53	0.70	1.05
Karate		0.44	0.70	1.05
Kayaking		0.53	0.70	0.96
7.8 mph (12.5 kph)	0.68		
9.4 mph (15.0 kph)	0.96		
Lacrosse		0.53	0.70	0.88
Modern dancing		0.44	0.53	0.70
Mountaineering		0.61	0.70	0.88
Orienteering		0.70	0.88	1.05
Racquetball		0.53	0.79	1.05
Rebounding		0.31	0.44	0.53
Rollerskating		0.44	0.57	0.70
Rope skipping		0.61	0.88	1.05
66 per min	0.86		
84 per min	0.92		
100 per min	0.96		
120 per min	1.00		
125 per min	1.02		
130 per min	1.03		
135 per min	1.05		
145 per min	1.06		
Rowing		0.61	0.88	1.14
2.5 mph (4 kph)	.48		
5.0 mph (8 kph)	0.90		
7.5 mph (12 kph)	1.18		
10.0 mph (16 kph)	1.44		
12.5 mph (20 kph)	1.67		

	Health points per minute		
	Intensity*		
Activity	Light	Moderate	Heavy
Rugby	0.53	0.70	0.96
Scuba diving	0.35	0.44	0.53
Sculling	0.35	0.53	0.88
Skateboarding	0.44	0.57	0.70
Skating (ice)	0.35	0.61	1.14
11.3 mph (18 kph) 0.35			
15.6 mph (25 kph) 0.42			
17.5 mph (28 kph) 0.81			
20.0 mph (32 kph) 0.95			
22.5 mph (36 kph) 1.33			
Snorkeling	0.35	0.44	0.53
Soccer	0.44	0.61	0.96
Softball	0.26	0.35	0.44
Squash	0.53	0.79	1.05
Stair climbing	0.35	0.61	0.96
Swimming (beach)	0.18	0.26	0.35
Swimming (pool)	0.26	0.44	0.79
1.3 mph (2 kph) 0.38			
1.6 mph (2.5 kph) 0.60			
1.9 mph (3.0 kph) 0.78			
2.2 mph (3.5 kph) 1.01			
2.5 mph (4.0 kph) 1.19			
Synchronized swimming	0.35	0.53	0.70
Table tennis	0.26	0.44	0.70
Tennis	0.35	0.53	0.88
Volleyball	0.44	0.53	0.70
Walking up stairs	0.35	0.53	0.70
Water polo	0.53	0.70	0.96
Wrestling	0.53	0.79	1.05

*Light intensity results in minimal perspiration and only a slight increase in breathing above normal (RPE of less than 12). Moderate intensity results in definite perspiration and above normal breathing (RPE of 12-13). Heavy intensity corresponds to heavy perspiration and breathing (RPE of more than 13). These values are adapted from an expert committee report of the Canada Fitness Survey - source M. Jette et al., Clinical Cardiology, 13 (1990): 555-565.

Chapter 4
Prescription

❏ If you're a novice exerciser, consider using one of my beginning exercise programs (see chapter 3). Let your doctor help you adapt it to suit the medical realities of your particular case of arthritis.

❏ Use our Health Points System if you have mild or no joint pain and inflammation and your functional capacity is not too severely limited by your arthritis.

❏ Don't use our Health Points System if you are suffering a severe arthritis flare-up, have severe symptoms in many joints most of the time, or if your functional capacity is severely limited by joint damage/deformity/instability or other arthritis complications.

❏ When using our Health Points System, modulate your frequency, intensity, and duration of exercise to earn 50 to 100 points each week.

❏ Do not attempt to earn your quota of health points in fewer than 3 workouts—on at least 3 separate days—each week.

❏ Keep your goals realistic and modify them continually as your condition changes.

❏ If your condition is such that you cannot attain the desired weekly number of health points, don't become discouraged. Provided you perform some type of aerobic exercise for a minimum of 15 minutes at least 3 days a week, you'll derive important health benefits.

Chapter 5

Staying Within the Safe-Exercise Zone: Essential Guidelines for People With Arthritis

F ortunately, much of the guesswork has disappeared from the process of prescribing exercise as a form of arthritis therapy. Well-informed physicians can prescribe exercise just as they would medications. However, as in the case of drugs, certain precautions must be taken to make sure your exercise regimen is both safe and effective.

Even people without arthritis who are involved in an exercise program should adhere to certain general safety guidelines, detailed in other books from the Cooper Clinic, such as *Running Without Fear*,[1] *The Aerobics Program for Total Well-Being*,[2] and *The New Aerobics for Women*.[3] Rather than repeat all these general precautions here, I want to focus on the special problems and hazards associated with exercise for arthritis patients.

NINE SAFE-EXERCISE GUIDELINES

The safety guidelines below are intended to reduce the chances that exercise will exacerbate your arthritis condition or make worse any systemic complications you already have. Moreover, these directives will help prevent exercise-related cardiac complications and musculoskeletal injuries. I urge you to follow them and listen to the advice of your doctor.

EXERCISE SAFETY GUIDELINE 1

Have a thorough medical evaluation before starting your exercise program—and at regular intervals thereafter.

All arthritis patients should undergo a complete medical exam and obtain their doctor's permission before they embark on an exercise program. The only people excused from an exam are those with mild arthritis who can place a checkmark next to every one of these statements:

✓ Foregoing a Medical Exam ✓

_____ I have complete functional capacity with the ability to carry on all of the usual duties of everyday life without handicaps (that is, functional capacity class 1 in the box on page 15).

_____ My arthritis is localized in joints that won't be used during the form of exercise I choose to do. (See page 107.)

_____ I have a type of arthritis that isn't associated with systemic complications.

_____ I have no more than one major coronary artery disease risk factor. These risk factors are

- high blood pressure (i.e., on at least two occasions, systolic blood pressure above 159 mmHg or diastolic blood pressure above 89 mmHg; *or* I'm taking hypertension medication);
- a blood cholesterol level above 239 mg/dl (6.18 mmol/L);
- cigarette smoking;
- diabetes; and

- a family history of coronary artery disease or other athero-sclerotic disease (parents or siblings had it before age 55).

_____ I have no symptoms suggestive of cardiovascular disease, such as pain or discomfort in the chest that is brought on or worsened by exercise.

_____ I have no known chronic diseases other than arthritis.

_____ I'm under age 40 (if male) or 50 (if female).

Most of you will probably be candidates for a medical screening. For what to expect in a thorough arthritis pre-exercise screening exam, see Appendix B.

For certain arthritis sufferers, the risks of exercise may outweigh the benefits. Your doctor's permission to exercise will depend primarily on the type and severity of your arthritis, and whether systemic complications or other chronic diseases pose a threat. If your physician finds any of the following conditions during your exam, you should avoid aerobic exercise until therapy or the passage of time controls or corrects the condition.

✓ Do *Not* Exercise if Your Physician ✓ Indicates You Have Any of These Conditions

_____ Unstable angina pectoris or a recent severe heart attack

_____ Recent significant change in my resting ECG that has not been adequately investigated

_____ A recent embolism

_____ Thrombophlebitis or an intracardiac thrombus

_____ Active or suspected myocarditis or pericarditis

_____ Acute or inadequately controlled heart failure

_____ Moderate to severe aortic stenosis

_____ Clinically significant hypertrophic obstructive cardiomyopathy

_____ Suspected or known aneurysm—cardiac or vascular—that my physician feels may be worsened by exercise

_____ Uncontrolled arrhythmias that are considered to be clinically significant

(Cont.)

_____ Resting heart rate greater than 120 beats per minute

_____ Third-degree heart block

_____ Uncontrolled hypertension with resting systolic blood pressure above 200 mmHg or diastolic blood pressure above 120 mmHg

_____ Recent fall in systolic blood pressure of more than 20 mmHg that was not caused by medication

_____ Uncontrolled metabolic disease, such as diabetes mellitus, thyrotoxicosis, or myxedema

_____ Acute infection

_____ Fever (oral temperature of 99.5 °F [37.5 °C] or above)

_____ Chronic infectious disease—such as mononucleosis, hepatitis, or AIDS—that my doctor feels may be worsened by exercise

_____ Significant electrolyte disturbances

_____ Major emotional distress (psychosis)

_____ Neuromuscular or musculoskeletal disorders that may be worsened by exercise in my physician's opinion

_____ Pregnancy complications

_____ Any other condition known to preclude exercise

Note. From American College of Sports Medicine: Guidelines for Exercise Testing and Prescription, 4th edition. Philadelphia, Lea and Febiger, 1991. Adapted with permission.

Your pre-exercise medical exam won't be your last. Periodic checkups are important because arthritis is a progressive disease; new complications may develop or existing ones may worsen. The course that your arthritis takes cannot be predicted. Nor can anyone guess the exact impact that regular exercise will have on your body.

The central principle of arthritis rehabilitation is this: Therapeutic decisions must be continually modified based on each patient's response to them. That's why I think an evaluation after 12 weeks on an exercise program is important. It gives your physician the opportunity to alter your exercise regimen, if necessary, or any other problematic aspects of your therapy. Besides a physical examination and the verbal information you give to your doctor in answer to questions, this follow-up exam ideally should include a re-assessment of your range of motion, strength, and aerobic fitness. Further X rays and other tests are left to your doctor's judgment.

Provided no disturbing abnormalities are detected, exercise-related checkups can be annual thereafter. However, should you notice disturbing symptoms at any time between regularly scheduled doctor visits, do not hesitate to get an immediate appointment to have them looked into.

EXERCISE SAFETY GUIDELINE 2

Find out whether you need direct medical supervision when you exercise—and whether it's only during the early weeks of the program or on a permanent basis.

Just about everyone with arthritis is capable of doing carefully tailored range-of-motion and muscle-strengthening exercises. But for selected arthritis patients, aerobic exercise may be too risky. For other arthritis patients, aerobic exercise may be possible—*but only under special supervised conditions.* A "medically supervised" exercise program is one in which a doctor or other appropriately qualified health professional—such as a physical therapist, exercise physiologist, or nurse—is present and overseeing the exercise. If you meet any of the following conditions, you should err on the side of caution and begin exercising in a supervised program, at least for the first 12 weeks.

✓   **Conditions That Require**   ✓
Supervised Exercise

_____ My arthritis limits my functional capacity to the point where I fall into class 3 (see the box on page 15).

_____ I have a history of joint surgery due to arthritis.

_____ My arthritis is of a type and severity where my heart, lungs, blood vessels, or nervous system is now involved.

(Cont.)

_____ I have another disease or condition that makes aerobics problematic because it predisposes me to exercise-related complications. Examples of such conditions are coronary artery disease; chronic bronchitis or emphysema; peripheral vascular disease; severe kidney disease; diabetes; cancer; or extreme obesity.

To find a medically supervised exercise program, ask your doctor or the local branch of the Arthritis Foundation if you live in the United States. A local cardiac rehabilitation program is a good choice because they are aimed at patients, such as yourself, with special medical needs.

EXERCISE SAFETY GUIDELINE 3

Be thoroughly versed in the warning signs of an impending cardiac complication.

The information I'm giving you about exercise safety is not meant to scare you away. The fact remains that exercise is a far more normal state of human affairs than indolence and it can be done with a great degree of confidence by most people with arthritis.

What it comes down to is this: You're probably far more likely to die from the deleterious effects of sedentary living than you are to suffer from sudden death during exercise. On the other hand, it's still prudent to keep your risk as low as reasonably possible. One of the best ways to boost your risk-to-benefit ratio is to remember this axiom:

Although death during exercise is always unexpected, it's seldom unheralded.

In other words, in most instances, you'll have some warning that things are awry. The box on page 103 lists the bodily signs indicating that all might not be well with your heart. Should you experience any of them before, during, or just after your exercise sessions, discuss them with your doctor before continuing with exercise.

WARNING SIGNS OF HEART PROBLEMS

✓ *Pain or discomfort in your chest, abdomen, back, neck, jaw, or arms.* Such symptoms may be signs of an inadequate supply of blood and oxygen to your heart muscle because of potentially serious conditions such as atherosclerotic plaque buildup in your coronary arteries.

✓ *A nauseous sensation during or after exercise.* This can result from a variety of causes, but it can also signify a cardiac abnormality.

✓ *Unaccustomed shortness of breath during exercise.* Any kind of aerobic exercise may make you huff and puff. This isn't what I'm referring to here. Let's say an ordinary part of your routine is to walk 2 miles (3.2 kilometers) in 35 minutes with no breathlessness. If one day you can't do it anymore, you should be alarmed.

✓ *Dizziness or fainting.* This can occur in perfectly healthy people who don't follow proper exercise protocol and fail to cool down adequately. Anyone could feel dizzy momentarily or even actually faint if he or she stops exercising suddenly. The type of dizziness I'm concerned about occurs while you're exercising rather than upon stopping suddenly. This is a more probable sign of a serious heart problem and warrants immediate medical consultation.

✓ *An irregular pulse, particularly when it's been regular in your past exercise sessions.* If you notice what appears to be extra heartbeats or skipped beats, notify your doctor. This too might not be anything of significance; on the other hand, it could point to heart problems.

✓ *A very rapid heart rate at rest.* This means 100 beats per minute or higher after at least 5 minutes of rest. Although this could result from a variety of causes, including a fever, it can also point to cardiac abnormalities. It should be reported to your doctor.

EXERCISE SAFETY GUIDELINE 4

Put safety at the top of your exercise priority list by following proper exercise protocol.

When it comes to exercise, there's a right way and a wrong way to do it, a safe way and a dangerous way. Even people without arthritis who exercise should adhere to certain general safety guidelines, all of which have been described in detail in other books from the Cooper Clinic. Those included here have special relevance for exercisers with arthritis:

• *Warm up and cool down adequately—a minimum of 5 minutes for each.* Over 70% of all cardiac problems that surface during exercise do so either at the beginning or end of a session, and are thought to be related to inadequate warming-up or cooling-down. Also, warming up may reduce your risk for injuries.

• *Don't exercise in adverse climatic conditions, particularly without taking adequate precautions.* Hyperthermia—an overheating of the body during exercise—impairs your ability to exercise and predisposes you to heat stroke, a potentially fatal condition. The symptoms of hyperthermia include headache, dizziness, confusion, stumbling, nausea, cramps, and cessation of sweating or excessive sweating.

To avoid hyperthermia, here are four preventive measures you can take:

—If you're exercising outdoors, let weather conditions be your guide to the amount and intensity of exercise you should indulge in on a given day. When heat and humidity are high,

Symptoms of hyperthermia

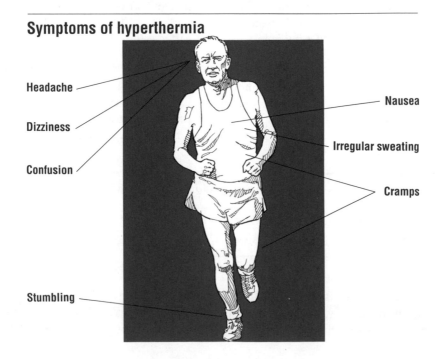

Headache

Dizziness

Confusion

Nausea

Irregular sweating

Cramps

Stumbling

be sensible. Don't engage in strenuous exercise. Likewise, be aware that cold weather worsens the usual disease symptoms in some people with arthritis. If this is so for you, you may need to modify your exercise program accordingly on such days.[4]

—Drink fluids while you're exercising, especially on hot days. Do this even if you're not thirsty. About 15 minutes before you begin your session, drink about 8 ounces (or 240 ml) of cold water, which is absorbed more quickly than tepid. If your workout lasts longer than 30 minutes, take another 8-ounce drink at 15 to 20-minute intervals during exercise.

—When exercising in warm weather, wear clothing that promotes heat loss. Fabrics that "breathe," such as a mesh or "fishnet" T-shirt, are good choices.

—If you must exercise in the heat, sponge off the exposed parts of your body with cool water at regular intervals.

• *Skip exercise when you have a fever, influenza, or other moderately serious acute illness.* You may not think it's necessary to include this warning. After all, who would want to exercise when they're sick? Believe it or not, lots of diehards I know would.

Certain types of arthritis may sometimes be accompanied by fever; rheumatoid arthritis is one of them. In such cases, the fever is usually the result of an infection, but sometimes the fever has no obvious explicable cause. *If your fever is due to infection, avoid strenuous aerobic exercise until your body temperature has returned to normal for at least 24 hours.* (I do not include gentle range-of-motion exercises in this admonition.)

Why are an infectious fever and aerobics a bad combination? Because heavy exertion coupled with an infection—including influenza—can trigger hyperthermia, worsen the infection, and sometimes place you at risk for a potentially lethal inflammatory condition of the heart muscle called *viral myocarditis.*[5]

On the other hand, if you have a fever but your doctor has assured you that it's not caused by an infection, you can undertake aerobics provided your oral temperature isn't 99.5 °F (37.5 °C) or above and you adhere closely to the recommendations for the prevention of hyperthermia (see page 104).

Acute illnesses usually subside on their own after a relatively short time or can be cured. If you've got nothing more serious than a cold, go ahead with aerobics if your temperature is normal and you feel like it. But when your acute ailment is more serious—and especially if it's accompanied by fever—sit out all forms of strenuous exercise until you're better. After an illness, ease back into aerobics gradually over the course of at least a week or two.

• *Wear quality shoes designed for the activity you're doing.* The right shoes are crucial for anyone, especially one with arthritis, who wants to avoid foot and knee problems and injuries. Because of recent technological advances, there are shoes specially designed for particular weight-bearing activities, and they are engineered to suit different types of feet. A qualified health professional is the best source of information about shoes to meet your particular needs. I'd also suggest that you patronize a quality shoe store where the sales staff are knowledgeable about athletic footgear. If you're a jogger, consult the periodic shoe evaluations that appear in the various runners' magazines. These consumer guides give you a look at the choices in various categories of athletic footgear and highlight what to seek out and what to avoid.

On a similar note, you should always try to perform any high-impact, weight-bearing activity, such as jogging, on a soft rather than a hard, resistant surface. Choose grass over cement, for example. And when it comes to preventing injuries, be aware that the most common cause of musculoskeletal injuries is performing too much exercise too soon!

EXERCISE SAFETY GUIDELINE 5

Choose forms of aerobic exercise that minimize the stress on painful, damaged, or deformed joints.

Which aerobic exercise you choose should depend largely on the location of your arthritis. Stick with exercises that place minimum stress on your affected joints. By consulting Table 5.1, for example, people with osteoarthritis of their knees or hips, who are doing weight-bearing forms of exercise that cause them moderate to severe pain, would discover that swimming, aqua-aerobics, or arm-cycle ergometry are better choices because they're much less likely to trigger pain in their problem joints. Reducing the intensity at which you perform a specific exercise is another way to reduce the amount of stress on joints.

Table 5.1
Joints Stressed by Aerobic Activities

Aerobic activity	Joints stressed						
	Ankle	Knee	Hip	Shoulder	Elbow	Wrist	Spine
Walking	+	+	+	—	—	—	+
Jogging	++	++	++	—	—	—	++
Stationary cycling (legs only)	+/—	+	+	—	—	—	+/—
Stationary cycling (arms and legs)	+/—	+	+	+/—	+/—	+/—	+/—
Arm cycle ergometry	—	—	—	+	+	+	+/—
Outdoor cycling	+/—	+	+	+/—	+/—	+/—	+/—
Swimming	—	—	—	+/—	+/—	—	+/—
Aqua-aerobics	+/—	+/—	+/—	+/—	+/—	—	+/—
Cross-country skiing machines	+/—	+/—	+	+/—	+/—	+/—	+
Stair-climbing machines	++	++	++	+/—	—	—	+
Rope skipping	++	++	++	+/—	+/—	+	++
Rebounding	+/—	+/—	+/—	—	—	—	—
Aerobic dance (high-impact)	++	++	++	+	+	+	++
Aerobic dance (low-impact)	+	+	+	+	+	+	+
Bench aerobics	++	++	++	+	+	+	+

Note. Adapted from "Arthritis and Aerobic Exercise: A Review" by R.W. Ike, 1989, *Physician and Sportsmedicine, 17,* pp. 128-139.

++ = High stress; + = moderate stress; +/— = mild stress; — = no significant stress.

The most popular aerobic exercises among our arthritis patients are walking, swimming, aqua-aerobics, and cycling. This does not rule out other choices, such as jogging, rebounding (running in place on a trampoline), aerobic dance, and certain recreational sports. Find the options that work best with your condition.

EXERCISE SAFETY GUIDELINE 6

Know the extent of your joint inflammation and pain—and how exercise is affecting them.

In other words, *stay in tune with your body*. This is critical because many types of arthritis, especially rheumatoid, tend to fluctuate. In periods of remission, the pain and inflammation may be slight. But during flare-ups, when pain is severe, you may have to cut back drastically on your exercise regimen. Monitor your arthritis inflammation by taking note of any obvious symptoms. To recap, the inflammatory symptoms and signs are *joint pain, tenderness, swelling, warmth, and redness*.

You should be aware that making judgments about your condition based on some symptoms or signs—especially swelling—can be somewhat misleading. For example, there's a distinction between a bony swelling resulting from bone overgrowth and swellings from other causes. The swelling of soft tissues around a joint or any swelling due to excess fluid build-up inside the joint space (known as an "effusion") are both signs of active arthritic inflammation. A bony overgrowth is not. How do you know which you have? Swelling from a bony overgrowth will feel very hard to the touch, whereas soft-tissue swelling and effusions generally won't. If you're in any doubt whatsoever, ask your doctor.

Pain is the most common symptom those with arthritis experience. Although it does not necessarily result from inflammation, pain is a good cautionary indicator. The pain rating scale on page 109 will help you stay within your individual safe-exercise zone during every workout.

Before each exercise session, use the scale to evaluate the extent of your overall joint pain and each painful joint. If any of your joints are warm to the touch, red, or swollen (for reasons other than a bony overgrowth), or if you have a pain rating of 30 or above in any joint, *you must not exercise those joints vigorously during your workout*. Certain low-intensity aerobic exercises that don't put much stress on an involved joint may still be possible. In general, such symptoms don't preclude range-of-motion exercises to prevent the development of contractures or some isometric muscle-strengthening exercises.

During your workouts, don't push yourself to where your pain rating increases by more than 10 points. Should this occur, immediately reduce your exercise intensity or switch to another activity that does not involve your painful joints. After each exercise session, use the scale to determine how your workout has affected your joint pain in general. (Be sure to make the distinction between aching muscles, which many novice exercisers experience, and joint pain.) If your

Arthritis Pain Rating Scale

No pain | 5 15 25 35 45 55 65 75 85 95 | **Intense pain—as bad as it could be**

10 20 30 40 50 60 70 80 90

0   **Moderate**   100
            pain

Rate your pain:

_____ Overall rating *before* your exercise session*

Pain in specific joints beforehand:

_____	*Foot/toes*	_____	*Hand/fingers*
_____	*Ankle*	_____	*Wrist*
_____	*Knee*	_____	*Elbow*
_____	*Hip*	_____	*Shoulder*
_____	*Spine*	_____	*Other*

_____ Overall rating *immediately after* your exercise session*

_____ Overall rating *two hours after* your exercise session*

*Transfer the ratings to the Exercise Log on page 63.

---

overall joint pain is worse at the end of the workout, wait 2 hours and rate your joint pain again. If it's still more intense than it was before your workout, you're overdoing it. The conclusion is unequivocal: *You need to change your exercise regimen.*

EXERCISE SAFETY GUIDELINE 7

Never disregard a trend indicating that your functional capacity is deteriorating or your symptoms—in the form of pain and/or inflammation—are getting worse.

The comparison of various blood tests, such as your ESR (see Appendix B), done over time will always be the most accurate way to assess inflammation, but who has the financial resources or time to have them done constantly? In place of them, I recommend that you track the long-term course of your arthritis via our pain rating scale (page 109) and Appendix C, a "Functional Capacity Scorecard" developed at Stanford University. Recording your pain ratings in your daily training log and filling in the scorecard monthly will help you and your doctor see at a glance how you're doing. If you note a trend indicating an improvement in your condition, be happy and continue your exercise program. If you detect a trend in the other direction, a change in your regimen is warranted.

EXERCISE SAFETY GUIDELINE 8

Do not engage in passive forms of exercise unless you've received specific instructions from a qualified health professional outlining how to do it.

There are three kinds of range-of-motion and stretching exercises— "passive," "active," and "active-assisted." You're engaging in a passive exercise when someone else is guiding your joint through its range of motion while you relax and don't actively help by contracting your muscles. For people with arthritis whose joint motion may be constrained, this type of exercise is not a good idea, unless performed by an appropriate health professional, and can be very painful.

In active exercise you contract your muscles to propel movement. Active-assisted exercises are a hybrid of the two. You're activating your muscles to move a joint through its range of motion but with assistance from someone. Active-assisted exercises can also be done by using one part of your body (for example, your right arm) to foster a range-of-motion movement in another part of your body (your left shoulder).

The risk of injury or of exacerbating your arthritis is far higher with passive and even active-assisted exercises than with active ones. That's why the programs in this book emphasize active range-of-motion and stretching exercises. Only do passive or active-assisted exercises when a physical therapist or other qualified health professional has cleared you to do so—or is the one doing the assisting.

Types of range-of-motion & stretching exercises

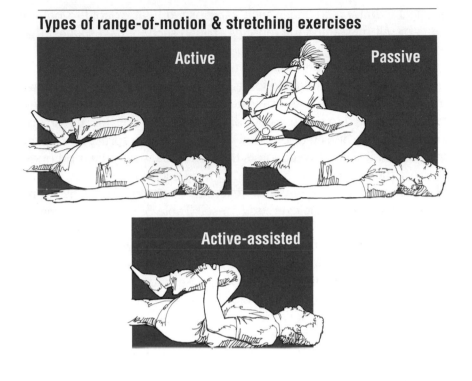

EXERCISE SAFETY GUIDELINE 9

If you're taking a prescribed anti-inflammatory medication, choose a time of day to exercise when the drug will be exerting its greatest influence and your joint pain and stiffness will be at a minimum.

For medications taken 4 times a day, this will be, in most people, 30 minutes to 2 hours after you took the drug. For medications taken on a 3-times daily schedule, it will more likely be 1 to 3 hours after ingestion. And for once or twice daily medication, figure 1 to 6 hours later.

On the other hand, I don't want you to create a situation where you specifically take a painkiller to help you through a workout, whether it's a prescribed medication or an over-the-counter drug. Pain is an expressive symptom. You must always be in a position to "hear" your body when it's telling you to slow down. Rather than relying on painkillers to get through a workout, arthritis patients should use physical therapy techniques such as applying heat or cold to painful joints or self-massaging the muscles around such joints. I suggest that you discuss these options with your doctor.

Some arthritis patients have corticosteroid anti-inflammatory drugs injected directly into inflamed joints. If you're an exerciser, this "intra-articular" therapy has its drawbacks; it relieves pain so effectively you'll be tempted to overuse your diseased joints.[6] For this reason you should rest any injected joint for about 3 days before you resume normal use. If your injected joints happen to be weight-bearing ones, *stay off them for up to 3 weeks*. During such periods, you'll need to modify and de-intensify your exercise regimen. Avoid high and moderate stress aerobic exercise (consult Table 5.1, "Joints Stressed by Aerobic Activities" on page 107).

Rheumatoid arthritis patients are often treated with "disease-modifying anti-rheumatic drugs" (or DMARDs). Although these drugs have no obvious negative impact on exercise (and vice versa), a patient on DMARDs should probably avoid high-intensity exercises that raise his or her heart rate above 75% of its maximal value. Examples of DMARDs are hydroxychloroquine (Plaquenil), azathioprine (Imuran), methotrexate (Rheumatrex), auranofin (Ridaura), sulfasalazine (Aza-line, Azulfidine), penicillamine (Cuprimine, Depen), and gold sodium thiomalate (Myochrysine).

DRUG ALERT FOR ARTHRITIS PATIENTS

Ask your doctor if any medications you're taking place you at greater risk during exercise or modify your heart rate response to exercise.

EXERCISE SAFETY RECOMMENDATIONS SUMMARIZED

Table 5.2 enables you to see at a glance the type and frequency of exercise that is safe for you to do given the current status of your arthritis. It takes into account your level of pain, the presence of inflammatory signs, and your functional capacity as determined by the classification scheme on page 15. Persons in functional capacity class 3 must be sure to consult the final set of recommendations in this chart that are explicitly intended for them.

Table 5.2
Summary of Exercise Safety Recommendations:
Range-of-motion and stretching exercises
Muscle-strengthening exercises
Aerobic exercise

Mild arthritis pain (pain rating below 30)
and no other signs of inflammation

Range-of-motion and stretching exercises—Every day, do 3–5 repetitions of several
of the range-of-motion exercises shown in Figures 3.1–3.12. In addition and also
daily, do 1–3 repetitions of the flexibility stretching exercises shown in Figures
3.13–3.17.

Muscle-strengthening exercises—Three times a week on alternate days, do the
isotonic muscle-strengthening exercises shown in Figures 3.23–3.33. Perform 1
or 2 sets of each exercise, a set consisting of 8–16 repetitions.

Aerobic exercise—Each week, your goal is to earn 100 health points doing those
forms of aerobic exercises that do not exacerbate your arthritis.

Moderate arthritis pain (rating between 30 and 70)
and no other signs of inflammation

Range-of-motion and stretching exercises—Every day, do 3–5 repetitions of several
of the range-of-motion exercises shown in Figures 3.1–3.12. In addition and also
daily, do 1–3 repetitions of the flexibility stretching exercises shown in Figures
3.13–3.17.

Muscle-strengthening exercises—Work your unaffected joints doing the isotonic
exercises shown in Figures 3.23–3.33; 3 times a week on alternate days, perform
1 or 2 sets of each exercise, a set consisting of 8–16 repetitions. For affected
joints, do 2 or 3 repetitions daily of the isometric muscle-strengthening exercises
shown in Figures 3.18–3.22.

Aerobic exercise—Only if your lower-limb joints are the site of your moderate pain,
reduce your goal to earning over 50 health points. Otherwise, stick with 100 health
points. Be careful about the aerobic exercise you choose and, by all means, vary
your routine with cross- and interval training as described in chapter 3.

Severe arthritis pain (pain rating above 70)
and/or other signs of inflammation

Range-of-motion and stretching exercises
  • *Daily regimen for unaffected joints.* Every day, do 3–5 repetitions of several
    of the range-of-motion exercises shown in Figures 3.1–3.12. In addition, do
    1–3 repetitions of the stretching exercises shown in Figures 3.13–3.17.

(Cont.)

Table 5.2
(Continued)

Severe arthritis pain (pain rating above 70)
and/or other signs of inflammation

Range-of-motion and stretching exercises (Cont.)
- *Daily regimen for affected joints.* Gently perform 1 repetition of the range-of-motion and stretching exercises shown in Figures 3.1–3.12 and Figures 3.13–3.17.

Muscle-strengthening exercises
- *Isotonic regimen for unaffected joints.* Do the isotonic muscle-strengthening exercises in Figures 3.23–3.33. Three times a week on alternate days, perform 1 or 2 sets of each exercise, a set consisting of 8–16 repetitions.
- *Daily isometric regimen for affected joints.* Do only 1 repetition of the isometric exercises shown in Figures 3.18–3.22.

Aerobic exercise
- *You've got osteoarthritis or a similar type of arthritis with* **no systemic complications** *and either your arm or leg joints are affected—but not both.* If your lower-limb joints are your problem, be satisfied with earning over 50 health points instead of the usual 100; otherwise aim for 100 health points. Only engage in exercise that places mild or no stress on very painful or inflamed joints. Vary your routine with cross- and interval training (see chapter 3).
- *You've got rheumatoid arthritis or a similar type of arthritis* **with systemic complications** *and either your arm or leg joints are affected—but not both.* Try to do 15–30 minutes of aerobic exercise 3–5 days each week. Exercise at the lower end of your target heart rate zone, and do cross- and interval training. Choose exercises that place minimal stress on afflicted joints. The Health Points System is not specifically intended for you—but if you decide to use it, be satisfied with 50 points.
- *Your arms and legs are both severely affected by arthritis.* You'd be better off forgetting about a serious aerobics exercise program for now. If you're determined, however, make sure any aerobics you do is low in intensity and places only mild or no stress on affected joints. The Health Points System is not intended for you.

Functional capacity = class 3

Range-of-motion and stretching exercises—Provided your doctor has given you the necessary clearance, and depending on your current level of arthritis pain and inflammation, do these in accordance with the recommendations for Severe Arthritis Pain.

Functional capacity = class 3 (Cont.)

Muscle-strengthening exercises—Provided your doctor has given you the necessary clearance, and depending on your current level of arthritis pain and inflammation, do 1–3 repetitions each day of the isometric exercises shown in Figures 3.18–3.22. After at least 4 weeks on this program, consider including isotonic exercises (Figures 3.23–3.33) in accordance with the recommendations for Severe Arthritis Pain.

Aerobic exercise—Provided your doctor has given you the necessary clearance—and you are not too severely limited by your arthritis—aim for a minimum of 50 health points each week. If you are severely limited by your arthritis, ignore our Health Points System and aim simply for a minimum of 15 minutes of aerobic exercise 3–5 days each week. Choose exercises that place mild or no stress on involved joints. Make use of cross- and interval training. If you have severe arthritis pain (rating above 70) and/or other signs of inflammation, read the aerobic exercise guidelines for such persons in the preceding Severe Arthritis Pain section—if so indicated, do not use our health points or participate in a serious aerobics exercise program for now.

SOME CONCLUDING THOUGHTS

In this book, I've offered you a state-of-the-art method for using regular exercise to optimize both the quality and the quantity of your life. My advice has been based on what is currently known about exercise and arthritis. In years to come, more will certainly be learned about how arthritis patients such as yourself can derive the most from an exercise rehabilitation program. But you shouldn't wait until then to exercise your options and embark on a physically active lifestyle. Now is the time for you, in consultation with your doctor, to formulate your specific game plan from the prototypes I've provided.

The sooner you begin a sensible exercise program, the sooner you will reap the many rewards. Once you do get started, never forget that exercise should be fun. I've always enjoyed it thoroughly and have no doubt that with time you will too.

Good luck! And the best of health to you.

Chapter 5
Prescription

❐ Have a thorough medical evaluation before starting your exercise program—and at regular intervals thereafter.

☐ Find out whether you need direct medical supervision when you exercise—and over what period of time.

☐ Be thoroughly versed in the warning signs of an impending cardiac complication.

☐ Skip exercise when you have a fever, influenza, or other moderately serious acute illness.

☐ Don't perform too much exercise too early on in your program.

☐ Choose forms of aerobic exercise that minimize the stress on painful, inflamed, damaged, or deformed joints.

☐ Know the extent of your joint inflammation and pain—and how exercise is affecting them.

☐ If your joint pain is worse 2 hours after your workout than it was before, you need to alter your exercise regimen.

☐ Take your current level of arthritis pain, inflammatory symptoms, and functional capacity into account when setting exercise goals for yourself.

Appendix A

How to Take Your Pulse and Calculate Your Heart Rate

You have two pulse points to choose from—the radial artery in your wrist or the carotid artery in your throat. Your radial artery is the preferred place because the reading there is usually more accurate.

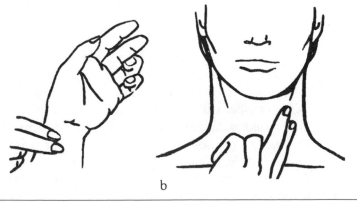

a   b

Figure A.1 Pulse points: a) radial artery, b) carotid artery. *Note.* From *ACSM Fitness Book* (p. 24) by The American College of Sports Medicine, 1992, Champaign, IL: Leisure Press. Copyright 1992 by The American College of Sports Medicine. Reprinted by permission.

Your two carotid arteries are located on either side of your windpipe. These arteries are large, and you should be able to locate them easily by gently pressing just to the right or left of your Adam's apple. But there are several things you must keep in mind. Don't press hard; press on only one carotid artery at a time; and do not press too near the jawbone. If you do any of these things your heart rate may slow down excessively and result in potentially harmful consequences, not to mention an inaccurate reading.

Taking your pulse is a three-step process. Here are instructions for taking a wrist pulse reading. Resort to your carotid artery only if you absolutely cannot locate the radial artery in your wrist.

1. *Locate the pulse in your wrist.* The hand of your wristwatch arm is the one you will use to monitor the pulse in your opposite wrist. Your "sensors" are the pads of your fingers, not your fingertips.

Place your index finger and middle finger at the base of the outer third of your wrist, the side on which your thumb is located. If you feel your wrist's tendons, you need to move your fingers further to the outside of your wrist. Do this incrementally, changing the location of your fingers by about a quarter of an inch until you finally locate a pulsation. Don't press too hard or you may obliterate your pulse. A light but firm pressure is all that is needed. You should be able to feel your pulse each time your heart beats, thus making your pulse rate equivalent to your heart rate.

2. *Count your pulse.* To determine your *resting heart rate*, count for 30 to 60 seconds. Your heart rate varies with your breathing; it slows down when you exhale and speeds up when you inhale. Thus if you count your pulse for shorter periods, you won't get a good average reading.

Taking a reading during exercise is different. Then your pulse rate is faster so a 10-second count is sufficient. If you're exercising in a stationary position—on a cycle ergometer, for example—you can count your pulse easily without stopping. However, if you're moving—such as walking or jogging—you'll need to stop, but not completely. Keep your legs moving while you take your pulse, which *you must do immediately*. If you wait for more than a second or two, your heart starts to slow down. This is true particularly if you are fit. If you count for longer than 10 seconds, you run the risk of greatly *underestimating* your heart rate.

When counting your pulse, count as "one" the first pulsation you feel *after* your watchhand hits a digit. Do *not* count as "one" any pulsation that occurs at the same time as the hand hits the digit. Continue the count until your watch registers 10 seconds. If a pulsation occurs at the same time as the watchhand hits the 10-second point, count it, but none thereafter.

3. *Calculate your heart rate.* After you've counted your pulse for 10 seconds, multiply that number by 6 to get your heart rate (beats per minute). Here's a chart with the calculations already done for 10-second pulse counts of 12 through 31:

12 = 72	17 = 102	22 = 132	27 = 162
13 = 78	18 = 108	23 = 138	28 = 168
14 = 84	19 = 114	24 = 144	29 = 174
15 = 90	20 = 120	25 = 150	30 = 180
16 = 96	21 = 126	26 = 156	31 = 186

Appendix B

Tests and Procedures in a Thorough Pre-Exercise Medical Exam

Here is a description of a state-of-the-art medical exam in a facility fully equipped for sophisticated testing. Your checkup may not be as comprehensive if the equipment isn't available or if your medical history indicates that your case doesn't warrant it.

✓   Checkup Checklist   ✓

_____ My physician or physician's assistant takes a thorough medical history. Its major purpose is to identify the diseases I know I have or any symptoms suggestive of disease and to document all the medications I'm currently taking. Among other things, it also covers my attitudes about exercise and arthritis in general and my ability to perform the physical activities of daily living.

I'm examined for other illnesses. In particular, I'm given a thorough cardiovascular exam, which includes the following:

_____ Measuring my blood pressure.

_____ Monitoring the pulses in my neck, arms, and legs.

_____ Listening to my neck, chest, heart, abdomen, and femoral arteries in my groin with a stethoscope.

_____ Inspecting the veins in my neck, examining my abdomen, and inspecting my ankles for any evidence of heart failure.

_____ Administering a blood-cholesterol test, if none was done recently. If the result this time is more than 200 mg/dl (5.17 mmol/L), a more detailed blood-lipid profile is ordered showing the ratio of the so-called good HDL-cholesterol to the bad LDL-cholesterol.

_____ Reading a resting electrocardiogram (ECG).

_____ Administering a treadmill exercise test (a "symptom-limited maximal exercise test") with ECG and blood pressure monitoring. This test is especially important if any of these conditions apply:

- I have any known or suspected cardiovascular disease, or two or more of the five major risk factors for it (see list in chapter 5, page 98);
- I have known or suspected lung disease;
- I'm a man over 40 years old;
- I'm a woman over 50 years old.

For any person with one or more of these conditions who is about to embark on an aerobic exercise program, this is the precautionary approach strongly recommended by the American College of Sports Medicine (ACSM). Though the ACSM has no specific recommendations for arthritis patients, I'd add that anyone with a type of arthritis associated with systemic manifestations should have a treadmill test, particularly if the person is over 30 years old or has had arthritis for more than 5 years.

_____ I'm checked for musculoskeletal problems and systemic arthritis complications.

_____ My body weight and, if possible, percentage body fat are measured.

_____ X rays are taken of the involved joints, especially if those X rays on file are over 1 year old. If I've had arthritis for more than 3 years and neck pain is one of the symptoms, my doctor should also take X rays of my neck (cervical) vertebrae.

_____ An ESR test is done. (This "erythrocyte sedimentation rate"—or "sed rate"—is a blood test that determines the overall amount of inflammation present in your body.) An ESR test is especially critical if I have the kind of arthritis associated with systemic complications.

_____ My hemoglobin is measured. A reduced hemoglobin concentration in the blood—known as "anemia"—sometimes develops in people with certain types of arthritis, including rheumatoid arthritis. Anemia impairs the body's ability to supply muscles with adequate oxygen during exercise.

_____ My joints are given range-of-motion and flexibility assessments of both the active and passive kind. An active evaluation means I move my joint through its full range of motion. A passive assessment means I remain relaxed and my doctor or physical therapist provides the locomotion to move my joint.

_____ My physician checks my body's muscular strength, with or without sophisticated equipment. Strength tests done with such equipment as a Cybex isokinetic dynamometer provide generally more objective and complete information.

_____ My physician exercises judgment in deciding what additional tests I need given my individual circumstances.

Appendix C

Functional Capacity Scorecard

How Much Does Arthritis Interfere With My Ability to Lead a Normal, Independent Life?

This functional capacity scoring system for arthritis patients was developed at Stanford University by Dr. James F. Fries. Make photocopies of this empty chart, for you should do this self-evaluation once a month.

I can do the following tasks (fill in score on line)	... without difficulty.	... with difficulty.	... with some help from someone else.	... I can't do it at all.
Dressing and Grooming				
Get my clothes out of the closet and drawers	0	1	2	3
Dress myself, including the handling of buttons, zipper, snaps, and so forth	0	1	2	3
Shampoo my hair	0	1	2	3
	Total	Total	Total	Total

Dressing/grooming total

(Cont.)

I can do the following tasks (fill in score on line)	... without difficulty.	... with difficulty.	... with some help from someone else.	... I can't do it at all.
Arising				
Stand up from a straight chair without using my arms for support	0	1	2	3
	Total	Total	Total	Total
				Arising total
Eating				
Cut the meat on my plate	0	1	2	3
Lift a full cup or glass to my mouth	0	1	2	3
	Total	Total	Total	Total
				Eating total
Walking				
Walk outdoors on flat ground	0	1	2	3
	Total	Total	Total	Total
				Walking total
Hygiene				
Wash and dry my entire body	0	1	2	3
Use the bathtub	0	1	2	3

I can do the following tasks (fill in score on line)	... without difficulty.	... with difficulty.	... with some help from someone else.	... I can't do it at all.
Hygiene (cont.)				
Turn faucets on and off	0	1	2	3
Get on and off the toilet	0	1	2	3
	Total	Total	Total	Total
				Hygiene total
Reaching				
Comb my hair	0	1	2	3
Reach for and get down a 5-pound bag of sugar that is above my head	0	1	2	3
	Total	Total	Total	Total
				Reaching total
Gripping				
Open push-button car doors	0	1	2	3
Open jars that have been previously opened	0	1	2	3
Use a pen or pencil	0	1	2	3
	Total	Total	Total	Total
				Gripping total

(Cont.)

I can do the following tasks (fill in score on line)	... without difficulty.	... with difficulty.	... with some help from someone else.	... I can't do it at all.
Outside activities				
Drive a car (if I drive at all)	0	1	2	3
Run errands and shop	0	1	2	3
	Total	Total	Total	Total

Outside activities total

Total for all 8 categories

Over the course of several months you'll be able to evaluate whether your functional capacity is improving or going downhill. If your scores are getting consistently worse, I suggest you talk to your doctor about altering your treatment program.

Note. From "Measurement of Patient Outcome in Arthritis" by J.F. Fries et al., 1980, *Arthritis and Rheumatism*, *23*, pp. 137-145. Adapted by permission of Lippincott and the author.

Notes

CHAPTER 1

[1]Duda, M. "King vs. Arthritis: Advantage, King." *Physician and Sportsmedicine* 17 (1989): 173-175.

[2]Altman, R.D. "Classification of Disease: Osteoarthritis." *Seminars in Arthritis and Rheumatism* 20 (1991): 40-47.

[3]Hamerman, D. "The Biology of Osteoarthritis." *New England Journal of Medicine* 320 (1989): 1322-1330.

[4]Ala-Kokko, L., et al. "Single Base Mutation in the Tyell Procollagen Gene (COL2A1) as a Cause of Primary Osteoarthritis Associated with a Mild Chondroplasia." *Proceedings of the National Academy of Science* 87 (1990): 6565-6568.

[5]Arthritis Foundation. *Practical Information: Where to Turn for Help*. Atlanta: Arthritis Foundation, 1989.

CHAPTER 2

[1]Leon, A.S., et al. "Leisure-Time Physical Activity Levels and Risk of Coronary Heart Disease and Death." *Journal of the American Medical Association* 258 (1987): 2388-2395.

[2]Samples, P. "Exercise Encouraged for People with Arthritis." *Physician and Sportsmedicine* 18 (1990): 123-126.

[3]Blair, S.N., et al. "Physical Fitness and All-Cause Mortality: A Prospective Study of Healthy Men and Women." *Journal of the American Medical Association* 262 (1989): 2395-2401.

[4]Powell, K.E., et al. "Physical Activity and the Incidence of Coronary Heart Disease." *Annual Review of Public Health* 8 (1987): 253-287.

[5]Blair, S.N., et al. "Physical Fitness and All-Cause Mortality: A Prospective Study of Healthy Men and Women." *Journal of the American Medical Association* 262 (1989): 2395-2401.

[6]Berlin, G.A., and Colditz, G.A. "A Meta-Analysis of Physical Activity in the Prevention of Coronary Heart Disease." *American Journal of Epidemiology* 132 (1990): 612-628.

[7]Reilly, P.A., et al. "Mortality and Survival in Rheumatoid Arthritis: A 25 Year Prospective Study of 100 Patients." *Annals of the Rheumatic Diseases* 49 (1990): 363-369.

[8]Pincus, T., Callahan, L.F., and Vaughn, W.K. "Questionnaire, Walking Time and Button Test Measures of Functional Capacity as Predictive Markers for Mortality in Rheumatoid Arthritis." *Journal of Rheumatology* 14 (1987): 240-251.

[9]Bouchard, C., et al., eds. *Exercise, Fitness, and Health. A Consensus of Current Knowledge.* Champaign, IL: Human Kinetics Publishers, 1990.

[10]Ekdahl, C., Anderson, S.I., and Svensson, B. "Muscle Function of the Lower Extremities in Rheumatoid Arthritis and Osteoarthritis." *Journal of Clinical Epidemiology* 42 (1989): 947-954.

[11]Kottke, F.J. "The Effects of Limitation of Activity Upon the Human Body." *Journal of the American Medical Association* 196 (1966): 825-830.

[12]Fisher, N.M., et al. "Muscle Rehabilitation: Its Effect on Muscular and Functional Performance of Patients with Knee Osteoarthritis." *Archives of Physical Medicine and Rehabilitation* 72 (1991): 367-374.

[13]Ike, R.W., Lampman, R.M., and Castor, C.W. "Arthritis and Aerobic Exercise: A Review." *Physician and Sportsmedicine* 17 (1989): 128-138.

[14]Fries, J.F. *Arthritis: A Comprehensive Guide to Understanding Your Arthritis.* Reading, MA: Addison-Wesley, 1989.

[15]Nordemar, R., et al. "Physical Training in Rheumatoid Arthritis: A Controlled Long-Term Study." *Scandinavian Journal of Rheumatology* 10 (1981): 17-23.

[16]Ekdahl, C., et al. "Dynamic Training and Circulating Levels of Corticotropin-Releasing Factor, Beta-Lipotropin and Beta-Endorphin in Rheumatoid Arthritis." *Pain* 40 (1990): 35-42.

[17]Semble, E.L., Loeser, R.F., and Wise, C.M. "Therapeutic Exercise for Rheumatoid Arthritis and Osteoarthritis." *Seminars in Arthritis and Rheumatism* 20 (1990): 32-40.

[18]Raglin, G.S. "Exercise and Mental Health. Beneficial and Detrimental Effects." *Sports Medicine* 9 (1990): 323-329.

[19]Ekblom, B., et al. "Effects of Short-Term Physical Training on Patients with Rheumatoid Arthritis." *Scandinavian Journal of Rheumatology* 4 (1975): 87-91.

[20]Thoren, P., et al. "Endorphins and Exercise: Physiological Mechanisms and Clinical Implications." *Medicine and Science in Sports and Exercise* 22 (1990): 417-428.

[21]Ekdahl, C., et al. "Dynamic Training and Circulating Levels of Corticotropin-Releasing Factor, Beta-Lipotropin and Beta-Endorphin in Rheumatoid Arthritis." *Pain* 40 (1990): 35-42.

[22]Yelin, E.H., and Felts, W.R. "A Summary of the Impact of Musculoskeletal Conditions in the United States." *Arthritis and Rheumatism* 33 (1990): 750-755.

[23]Arthritis Foundation. *Primer on the Rheumatic Diseases*, 9th ed. Atlanta: Arthritis Foundation, 1988.

[24]Thompson, P.D., et al. "Incidence of Death During Jogging in Rhode Island from 1975 through 1980." *Journal of the American Medical Association* 247 (1982): 2535-2538.

[25]Macera, C., et al. "Predicting Lower-Extremity Injuries Among Habitual Runners." *Archives of Internal Medicine* 149 (1989): 2561-2568.

[26]Walter, S., et al. "The Ontario Cohort Study of Running-Related Injuries." *Archives of Internal Medicine* 149 (1989): 2561-2564.

[27]Blair, S.N., Kohl, H.W., and Goodyear, N.N. "Rates and Risks for Running and Exercise Injuries: Studies in Three Populations." *Research Quarterly for Exercise and Sport* 58 (1987): 221-228.

CHAPTER 3

[1]Sapega, A.A., et al. "Biophysical Factors in Range-of-Motion Exercises." *Physician and Sportsmedicine* 9 (1981): 57-65.

[2]Gerber, L.H. "Rehabilitation of Patients With Rheumatic Diseases." In *Textbook of Rheumatology*, 3rd ed., edited by W.M. Kelly et al. Philadelphia: Saunders, 1989.

[3]Machover, S., and Sapecky, A.J. "Effects of Isometric Exercise on the Quadriceps Muscle in Patients with Rheumatoid Arthritis." *Archives of Physical Medicine and Rehabilitation* 11 (1966): 737-741.

[4]Fiatarone, M.A., et al. "High Intensity Strength Training in Nonagenarians. Effects in Skeletal Muscle." *Journal of the American Medical Association* 263 (1990): 3029-3034.

[5]Agre, J.C., et al. "Light Resistance and Stretching Exercise in Elderly Women: Effect Upon Strength." *Archives of Physical Medicine and Rehabilitation* 69 (1988): 273-276.

[6]Institute for Aerobics Research. *The Strength Connection*. Dallas: Institute for Aerobics Research, 1990.

[7]American College of Sports Medicine. "Position Stand. The Recommended Quantity and Quality of Exercise for Developing and Maintaining Cardiorespiratory and Muscular Fitness in Healthy Adults." *Medicine and Science in Sports and Exercise* 22 (1990): 265-274.

[8]Cooper, K.H. *Aerobics*. New York: Bantam Books, 1968.

[9]Blair, S.N., et al. "Exercise and Fitness in Childhood: Implications for a Lifetime of Health." In *Perspectives in Exercise Science and Sports Medicine*, edited by C.V. Gisolfi and D.R. Lamb. Vol. 2, *Youth, Exercise and Sport*. Indianapolis: Benchmark Press, 1989, 401-430.

[10]American Heart Association Medical/Scientific Statement. "Exercise Standards. A Statement for Health Professionals from the American Heart Association." *Circulation* 82 (1990): 2286-2322.

[11]Haskell, W.L., Montoye, H.J., and Orenstein, D. "Physical Activity and Exercise to Achieve Health-Related Physical Fitness Components." *Public Health Reports* 100 (1985): 202-212.

[12]Blair, S.N. *Living with Exercise*. Dallas: American Health Publishing Company, 1991.

[13]DeBusk, R.F., et al. "Training Effects of Long Versus Short Bouts of Exercise in Healthy Subjects." *American Journal of Cardiology* 65 (1990): 1010-1013.

[14]American College of Sports Medicine. "Position Stand. The Recommended Quantity and Quality of Exercise for Developing and Maintaining Cardiorespiratory and Muscular Fitness in Healthy Adults." *Medicine and Science in Sports and Exercise* 22 (1990): 265-274.

[15]American College of Sports Medicine. *Guidelines for Exercise Testing and Prescription*. Philadelphia: Lea & Febiger, 1991.

[16]Borg, G.A. "Psychophysical Bases of Perceived Exertion." *Medicine and Science in Sports and Exercise* 14 (1982): 377-387.

[17]Rippe, J.M., et al. "Walking for Health and Fitness." *Journal of the American Medical Association* 259 (1988): 2720-2724.

[18]Thomas, T.R., and Londeree, B.R. "Energy Cost During Prolonged Walking vs. Jogging Exercise." *Physician and Sportsmedicine* 17 (1989): 93-102.

[19]Yanker, G., and Burton, K. *Walking Medicine*. New York: McGraw-Hill, 1990.

[20]Nordemar, R., et al. "Physical Training in Rheumatoid Arthritis: A Controlled Long-Term Study." *Scandinavian Journal of Rheumatology* 10 (1981): 17-23.

CHAPTER 4

[1]Cooper, K.H. *The Aerobics Program for Total Well-Being*. New York: Bantam Books, 1982.

[2]Aponte, J. "A Swimming Program for Patients with Ankylosing Spondylitis." *Arthritis and Rheumatism* 30 (1987): S205.

[3]Koszuta, L.E. "Water Exercise Causes Ripples." *Physician and Sportsmedicine* 14 (1986): 163-167.

[4]Cooper, K.H. *Overcoming Hypertension*. New York: Bantam Books, 1990.

[5]Cooper, K.H. *Overcoming Hypertension*. New York: Bantam Books, 1990.

[6]Cooper, K.H. *The Aerobics Program for Total Well-Being*. New York: Bantam Books, 1982.

[7]DeBenedette, V. "Stair Machines: The Truth About This Fitness Fad." *Physician and Sportsmedicine* 18 (1990): 131-134.

[8]Gerberich, S.G., et al. "Analysis of the Acute Physiologic Effects of Minitrampoline Rebounding Exercise." *Journal of Cardiopulmonary Rehabilitation* 10 (1990): 395-400.

[9]Williams, C., and Gordon, N.F. "Bench Stepping. An At-Home Introduction to the Hottest Trend in Aerobics." *Shape* (April 1990): 96-101.

[10]Gordon, N.F., et al. "Effects of Rest Interval Duration on Cardiorespiratory Responses to Hydraulic Resistance Circuit Training." *Journal of Cardiopulmonary Rehabilitation* 9 (1989): 325-330.

[11]Paffenbarger, R.S., et al. "Physical Activity, All-Cause Mortality, and Longevity in College Alumni." *New England Journal of Medicine* 314 (1986): 605-613.

[12]Coyle, E.F. "Detraining and Retension of Training-Induced Adaptations." In *Resource Manual for Guidelines for Exercise Testing and Prescription*, edited by S.N. Blair et al. Philadelphia: Lea & Febiger, 1988.

CHAPTER 5

[1]Cooper, K.H. *Running Without Fear*. New York: Evans, 1985.

[2]Cooper, K.H. *The Aerobics Program for Total Well-Being*. New York: Bantam Books, 1982.

[3]Cooper, K.H., and Cooper, M. *The New Aerobics for Women*. New York: Bantam Books, 1988.

[4]Guedji, D., and Weinberger, A. "Effects of Weather Conditions on Rheumatic Patients." *Annals of the Rheumatic Diseases* 49 (1990): 164-169.

[5]Ilback, N-G., Fohlman, J., and Friman, G. "Exercise in Coxsackie B3 Myocarditis: Effects on Heart Lymphocyte Subpopulations and the Inflammatory Reaction." *American Heart Journal* 117 (1989): 1298-1302.

[6]Ekblom, B., and Nordemar, R., "Rheumatoid Arthritis," In *Exercise Testing and Exercise Prescription for Special Cases*, edited by J.S. Skinner. Philadelphia: Lea & Febiger, 1987.

Index